T0329857

Thank you for your purchase of
Facial Volumization: An Anatomic Approach!

Access your e-book now!

Scratch here to reveal your access code

How to redeem your code:

1. Create an account on Thieme's e-book store at ebookstore.thieme.com/register
2. Click the **My E-Books** link
3. Select **Redeem Access Code**
4. Enter this code to claim your e-book
5. You can now read your e-book online!

How to download your book for offline access:

On a compatible phone or tablet*:

1. Download the **Thieme Bookshelf** app from **iTunes** or **Google Play** after you've redeemed your access code
2. Validate your e-book store username and password
3. Select the e-book and tap to download it to your device
4. Your e-book is now available to read offline!

*This app is available for iPads and Android devices. The e-book cannot be downloaded to any apps or readers other than Thieme Bookshelf.

On your PC or Mac:

1. Download **iPublishCentral Reader**** from the e-book store after you've redeemed your access code: **ebookstore.thieme.com/downloadioffline**
2. Validate your e-book store username and password
3. Select the book and click to download
4. Your e-book is now available to read offline!

**You may need to download and install Adobe Air prior to downloading iPublishCentral. Instructions are on the link provided.

This code can only be redeemed one time. After redemption, it can be downloaded to multiple devices on your account.
An internet connection is required for initial access and download. This book cannot be returned if the code has been revealed.

For any questions, please visit ebookstore.thieme.com/faqs.

Connect with us on social media

Check out these techniques online
with videos on MediaCenter.Thieme.com!

	WINDOWS & MAC	TABLET
Recommended Browser(s)	Recent browser versions on all major platforms and any mobile operating system that supports HTML5 video playback. *All browsers should have JavaScript enabled.*	
Flash Player Plug-in	Flash Player 9 or higher. *For Mac users, ATI Rage 128 GPU doesn't support full-screen mode with hardware scaling.*	Tablet PCs with Android OS support Flash 10.1.
Recommended for optimal usage experience	Monitor resolutions: • Normal (4:3) 1024×768 or higher • Widescreen (16:9) 1280×720 or higher • Widescreen (16:10) 1440×900 or higher A high-speed internet connection (minimum 384 Kps) is suggested.	WiFi or cellular data connection is required.

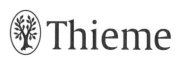

Facial Volumization

An Anatomic Approach

Jerome Paul Lamb, MD, FACS
Plastic Surgeon Diplomate of the American Board of Plastic Surgery, Inc.
Centerpoint Medical Center, Truman Medical Center
Independence, Missouri, United States

Christopher Chase Surek, DO
Chief Resident
Department of Plastic Surgery
University of Kansas Medical Center
Overland Park, Kansas, United States

58 illustrations

Thieme
New York • Stuttgart • Delhi • Rio de Janeiro

Executive Editor: Sue Hodgson
Developmental Editor: Jennifer Gann
Managing Editor: Elizabeth Palumbo
Director, Editorial Services: Mary Jo Casey
Production Editor: Torsten Scheihagen
International Production Director: Andreas Schabert
International Marketing Director: Fiona Henderson
International Sales Director: Louisa Turrell
Director of Sales, North America: Mike Roseman
Senior Vice President and Chief Operating Officer: Sarah Vanderbilt
President: Brian D. Scanlan
Medical Illustrator: Levent Efe

Library of Congress Cataloging-in-Publication Data

Names: Lamb, Jerome Paul, editor. | Surek, Christopher Chase, editor.
Title: Facial volumization : an anatomic approach / [edited by] Jerome Paul Lamb, MD, FACS, Plastic Surgeon Diplomate, American Board of Plastic Surgery, Inc., Centerpoint Medical Center, Truman Medical Center, Independence, Missouri, United States, Christopher Chase Surek, MD, Chief Resident, Department of Plastic Surgery, University of Kansas Medical Center, Overland Park, Kansas, United States.
Description: New York : Thieme, [2017]
Identifiers: LCCN 2017021388| ISBN 9781626236943 (print) | ISBN 9781626238640 (e-book)
Subjects: LCSH: Face--Surgery. | Surgery, Plastic.
Classification: LCC RD119.5.F33 F35 2017 | DDC 617.5/2059--dc23 LC record available at https://lccn.loc.gov/2017021388

This book is dedicated to those colleagues who have encouraged and mentored me along the way. Most notably, I thank Glenn Jelks, Bryan Mendelson, and Val Lambros, who saw the value of our preliminary research and encouraged us to publish. During my formative years, it was Don Kaminski, George Block, and Gus Colon who provided that guidance and support in medical school, general surgery, and plastic surgery residency that has graced my life. Lastly, this book is dedicated to my wife Carri, my son Jake, and my daughter Madi, who have given up time with me that will never be able to be returned in order for me to fulfill a dream.

Jerome Paul Lamb

I dedicate this book to those who have loved, supported, and inspired me. I want to thank my education mentors who have set great examples for me to follow. My true companion Krystle Surek, thank you for your patience during this process and for understanding my passion for this field. To Sharon Surek and Christopher L. Surek who raised me to chase my dreams and embodied the values of humility and unconditional love. To my grandfather Richard Weber who showed me that life is what you make of it and that giving up is never an option. Lastly, to our patients of past, present, and future—they are the instruments by which we are measured, and it is my sincere hope that this body of work will translate into renewed happiness and joy in their lives.

Christopher Chase Surek

Contents

Video Contents

Foreword

As a young plastic surgeon, I remember well how the interior of the face looked like a mysterious and dangerous territory where everything looked like everything else and only obedience to the empirical ritual of the facelift operation let me feel secure. In time, increasingly subtle changes of anatomy became old friends while passing them in surgery. I contemplated the retaining ligaments of the face—thin and weak individually, but very powerful in aggregate. Further along I began to understand how the anatomy contributed to both the look of the face and how such an understanding could be a tool to comprehending the older face and better ways to rehabilitate it. Knowledge is power.

In replacing or adding volume to the aging face subtleties of placement went from being ignored to being obvious. At first one is happy that an area can be filled at all. In time, one's powers of observation and discrimination increase to the point that earlier attempts look crude and artless and one sees and strives for more graceful and less exaggerated results.

Almost all aesthetic modifications of the face are based on anatomy, the details of which are usually the last consideration of the aesthetic practitioner. Facelifts were done for approximately 6 decades before the anatomy of the facial nerve was understood. The first several years of filler use was for the most part filling wrinkles. Injectors had very little understanding of the relationship of location and depth of placement to results until about a decade after their introduction when finally a more balanced and volumetric use of fillers was established. Cosmetic lasers were accepted very quickly before the occurrence of late depigmentation was appreciated. One might conclude that early commercial adoption of a technique precludes thoughtful study of its underlying science.

Things have changed: we have now grown into increased wisdom of many aspects of the face. The study of facial anatomy has blossomed in the last few years; with more attention being paid to areas of perceptual interest, the structures that define faces of different ages can be seen to have altered in knowable ways, not mysterious and arbitrary ones.

Drs. Lamb and Surek have given us a remarkable volume of facial anatomy, compiling information from other authors but also including extensive clean dissections and descriptions of their own. The greatest of explanatory tools, the diagrams, are particularly valuable as they are concise and correct and address the clinician's concerns. Anatomic phenomena of the face, hollows, ripples, mounds, and others are revealed to have their origins deep in the face in ways that are not intuitive. Treatments can be made more rationally with such understandings and many are included in this volume. Knowledge is power. This book is a major step forward in understanding not only the dry anatomy of the face, but how it works and how it can be modified for the good. Any student of the face will be well advised to study the topic and this book in particular.

Val Lambros, MD

Preface

Bryan Mendelson said it best: "Human beings are the only species on the planet whose age shows on their face." Treating the aging face is one of the great challenges of aesthetic surgery, and volume replenishment is a critical component of the treatment algorithm. Although volumization techniques are commonly performed, they are still relatively subjective, and they are often based on injector's "aesthetic eye." As anatomists and surgeons, we believe a strong knowledge of facial anatomy is critical for an injector to be accurate, safe, and consistent when performing facial volumization. Although there have been several published works about the individual components of the face, there has not been a comprehensive synthesis of facial anatomy specific to injection techniques. This book is designed to bridge the gap between the anatomy lab and your injection clinic. We intend to distill high-yield, clinically relevant anatomical details of commonly injected regions of the face and to guide the clinician in the safe conduct of these procedures.

The full-page illustrations will take the reader through each layer of the face, from deep to superficial, to demonstrate the scaffold construction of this complex anatomical landscape. As the reader turns the pages, they will arrive on new anatomical layers. On the left side of the page, the reader will find a written synopsis of the vascular, muscular, ligament, and adipose components of the specific layer paired with cadaveric photographs. Personally, we find the synergy between the anatomical descriptions and the medical illustration to equip us with a "snapshot" that we can think about when we are injecting these regions on our patients. It is our hope that this presentation improves your understanding of depth and of the plane of injection. At the end of Chapters 1, 2, and 4, we share our preferred techniques for volumization in each region; these descriptions are accompanied by a medical illustration depicting the critical anatomy for the defined technique.

The supplemental video companion of the book will take the reader step by step through each technique as it is performed on a patient. These videos contain medical illustrations in the top corner of the screen for the reader to visualize the anatomy as the injection is performed. The gliding nature and dynamic planes of the face create a formidable challenge for the injector when treating an aging face. Please consider this book as a companion, toolbox, and potential "secret weapon" to assist you with obtaining optimal aesthetic outcomes for your patients.

Jerome Paul Lamb and Christopher Chase Surek

Contributors

Mark Winter Ashton, MD
Professor
Department of Surgery
University of Melbourne
Parkville, Victoria, Australia

Jerome Paul Lamb, MD, FACS
Plastic Surgeon Diplomate of the American Board
   of Plastic Surgery, Inc.
Centerpoint Medical Center, Truman Medical
   Center
Independence, Missouri, United States

Sajna Shoukath, PhD
Student
Department of Surgery
University of Melbourne
Parkville, Victoria, Australia

Christopher Chase Surek, DO
Chief Resident
Department of Plastic Surgery
University of Kansas Medical Center
Overland Park, Kansas, United States

James D. Vargo, MD
Resident Physician
Department of Plastic Surgery
University of Kansas Medical Center
Kansas City, Missouri, United States

Chapter 1

The Midface

1 The Midface

Jerome Paul Lamb and Christopher Chase Surek

The Orbital Retaining Ligament, the Zygomaticocutaneous Ligaments, the Maxillary Retaining Ligaments, and the Masseteric Ligaments

The midface consists of both deep and superficial fat compartments along with two relevant anatomic spaces. The approach to the spaces and compartments has been previously published. The importance of hormonal receptors has been postulated but not investigated as a cause for midface descent, resulting in the aged appearance. Lambros postulated that midfacial aging was the result of volume loss rather than ligamentous or skin relaxation. Studies suggest a selective atrophy of deep fat compartments and relative hypertrophy of superficial fat, and this corresponds with larger adipocyte size in superficial fat compared to deep fat. The recent proposed concept of pseudoptosis or selective deflation of deep fat compartment leading to loss of support and sagging of the superficial cheek fat has led authors to advocate deep volumization techniques. We feel that the real decision lies in whether to inject in a sub-SMAS (subsuperficial muscular aponeurotic system) or supra-SMAS plane. This chapter will demonstrate the anatomy from deep to superficial portraying key anatomical targets for injection.

For the purpose of anatomical division, the midface can be divided into upper and lower regions by an imaginary topographic line traversing from the base of the alar crease to the superior tip of the tragus (**Fig. 1.1**). This line corresponds with the course of the zygomaticocutaneous retaining ligaments that arise from bone and insert onto skin (**Fig. 1.2**). This line acts as an equator between two distinctly different anatomical regions: the bone-supported cheek and the mobile cheek.

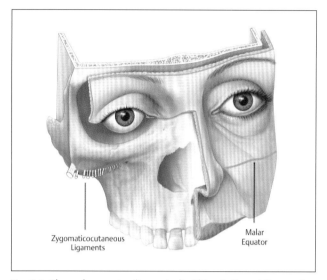

Fig. 1.1 The malar equator *(turquoise line)* bisects the midface and anatomically correlates with the zygomaticocutaneous ligaments.

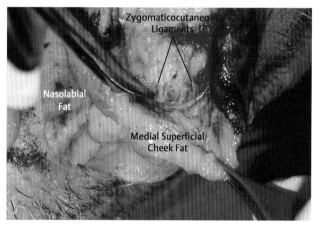

Fig. 1.2 The zygomaticocutaneous ligaments form the lower "hammock" border of the prezygomatic space. The ligaments serve as a partition of the upper and lower midface, respectively.

The Upper Midface

The orbital retaining ligament (ORL) is a bilaminar structure originating from the tear trough ligament. The ORL coalesces with the lateral orbital thickening as it traverses along the orbital aperture. The ORL separates the preseptal space from the prezygomatic space in the upper midface.

In addition to the zygomaticocutaneous ligaments, the main zygomatic ligament resides at the bony transition between the lateral and anterior midface at the maxillary deflection. As ligaments align with vascularized membranes, this region is clinically referred to as MacGregor's patch.

The Lower Midface

On the surface of the anterior maxilla reside the maxillary retaining ligaments. The clinical relevance will be discussed later in this chapter in correlation with the premaxillary space. Laterally, the upper and lower masseteric ligaments divide the "fixed SMAS" laterally from the "mobile SMAS" anteriorly.

Fig. 1.3 presents the gross anatomy of the ligaments discussed in this section.

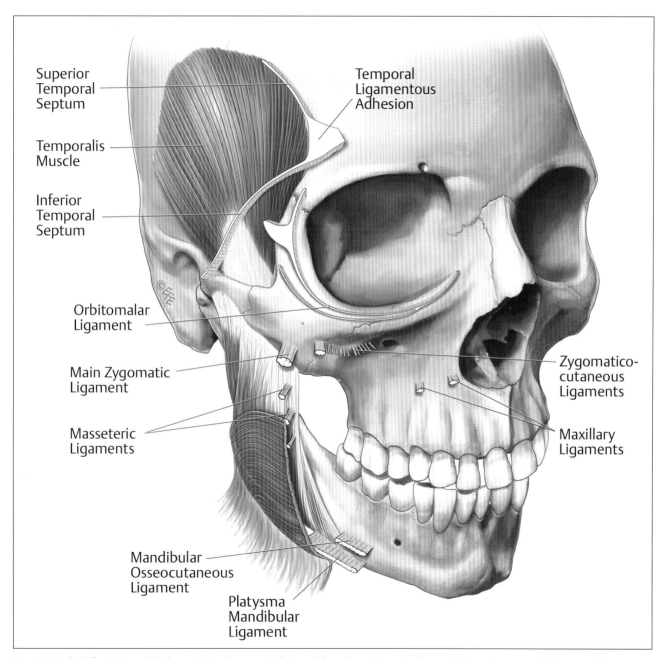

Fig. 1.3 Medical illustration of the key retaining ligaments of the midface: the orbitomalar ligament, the main zygomatic ligament, the zygomaticocutaneous ligaments, and the maxillary and masseteric ligaments.

The Preperiosteal Fat Pad and the Deep Pyriform Space

The Upper Midface

In the upper midface, deep to the orbicularis oculi, lie two layers of fat compartments: the preperiosteal fat compartment and the suborbicularis oculi fat compartment (SOOF), respectively. The SOOF will be discussed and demonstrated later in this chapter. However, deep to the SOOF and the prezygomatic space resides the preperiosteal fat compartment (**Fig. 1.4**). This fat is adherent to the bone of the maxilla and in cadaveric dissection is often noted to be covered with a dense fascia.

The Lower Midface

Deep on the anterior maxilla lies the deep pyriform space (**Fig. 1.5**). The deep pyriform space passes deep to the angular artery and abuts the recessing pyriform aperture (**Fig. 1.6**). We pos-tulate that, with age, the pyriform recesses, thereby enlarging the size of this space. In a cadaveric study, we found that the angular artery traverses lateral and superficial to the space and therefore is not preperiosteal at this level. This is an important finding for the injector as volumization in the deep pyriform space is not only effective in pyriform recess effacement, but also can be done safely without concern for intravascular compromise. Cannula pneumatization of the space demonstrates its deep connection to the upper midface through an undefined viaduct (**Video 1.1**). The lip elevators drape over this space as well, sending interlocking fibers into the nasolabial fold (**Fig. 1.7**). Volumization of this space may decrease the moment arm effect of these muscles on nasolabial fold elevation and efface-ment. The cephalic limitation of both the deep pyriform space and the premaxillary space is the tear trough ligament.

Fig. 1.8 presents the gross anatomy of the fat compartments and sub-SMAS spaces discussed in this section.

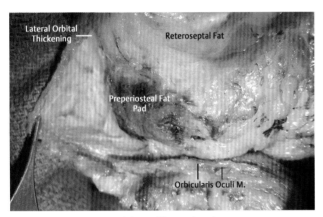

Fig. 1.4 The preperiosteal fat pad lies within the prezygomatic space adherent to the maxilla.

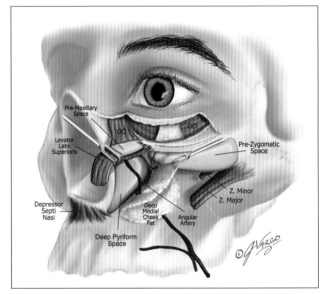

Fig. 1.5 Medical illustration of the deep pyriform space and impor-tant adjacent anatomical structures. (From Surek C, Vargo J, Lamb J. Deep pyriform space: anatomical clarifications and clinical implica-tions. Plast Reconstr Surg. 2016;138(1). 2016 with permission)

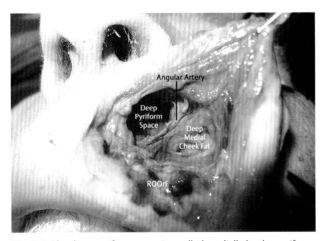

Fig. 1.6 The deep pyriform space is cradled medially by the pyriform aperture and depressor nasalis. The angular artery courses between the space and the deep medial cheek fat compartment. Note that the artery is not directly on periosteum, but superficial and lateral within the roof of the space. (From Surek C, Vargo J, Lamb J. Deep pyriform space: anatomical clarifications and clinical implications. Plast Reconstr Surg. 2016;138(1). 2016 with permission)

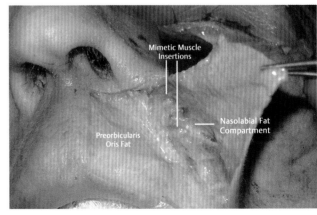

Fig. 1.7 Demonstration of the mimetic muscle insertions into the nasolabial fold. (From Surek C, Vargo J, Lamb J. Deep pyriform space: anatomical clarifications and clinical implications. Plast Reconstr Surg. 2016;138(1). 2016 with permission)

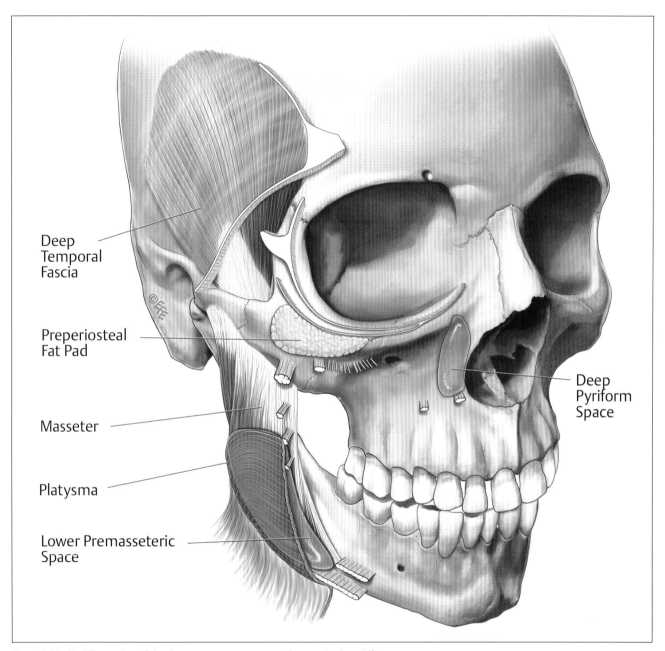

Fig. 1.8 Medical illustration of the deepest compartments and spaces in the midface.

Deep
Temporal
Fascia

Preperiosteal
Fat Pad

Masseter

Platysma

Lower Premasseteric
Space

Deep
Pyriform
Space

The Prezygomatic Space

The Upper Midface

Deep to the orbicularis oculi muscle, between the SOOF and the preperiosteal fat pad, lies the prezygomatic space (**Fig. 1.9**). The space is bounded superiorly by the ORL, which is synonymous with the orbitomalar ligament. The caudal extension of the space is limited by the zygomaticocutaneous ligaments. These ligaments act as a "hammock" network separating the upper midface from the lower midface. The lateral extent of the space is the lateral orbital thickening with a cephalic extension into the temporal tunnel.

On the floor of this space lies the preperiosteal fat. The investing fascia of SMAS on the posterior border of the orbicularis oculi is contiguous with the fascia overlying the preperiosteal fat compartment. The uniform construct of these structures forms a prezygomatic space capsule as described by Mendelson (**Fig. 1.10**). On blunt cannula access to this space from the lateral approach, the injector will use their opposite hand to "pinch and pull" the skin and orbicularis upward, allowing the cannula to pass deep and enter the prezygomatic space (**Fig. 1.11**; **Video 1.2**). Entrance into the space is confirmed by a palpable and audible penetration of the prezygomatic space capsule. The injector will feel and hear a "pop" once when they pass through the capsule into the space.

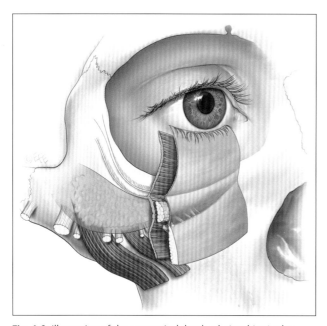

Fig. 1.9 Illustration of the anatomical depth relationships in the upper midface. The prezygomatic space is demonstrated in the deep suborbicularis plane (blue capsule). The orbitomalar ligament is demonstrated arborizing through the orbicularis oculi muscle inserting into the skin forming the tear trough crease. The zygomaticocutaneous ligaments arborize through the orbicularis, forming a partition between the infraorbital "malar" fat compartment superiorly and superficial cheek compartment inferiorly. The cutaneous insertion of the ligaments forms the characteristic skin crease demonstrated in clinical malar mounds.

For consistent deep volumization of the cheek, the prezygomatic space can be a secret weapon.

Fig. 1.12 depicts the gross anatomy of the prezygomatic space.

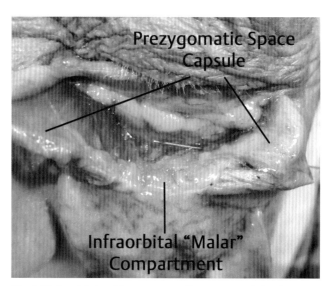

Fig. 1.10 Frontal view. The prezygomatic space capsule has been stained with methylene blue. The infraorbital "malar" fat compartment is noted superficial to the prezygomatic space and orbicularis oculi. Blunt cannulas placed percutaneously prior to dissection are found inside the prezygomatic space. (From Surek CC, Beut J, Stephens R, Jelks G, Lamb J. Pertinent anatomy and analysis for midface volumizing procedures. Plast Reconstr Surg 2015;135(5):818e–829e with permission).

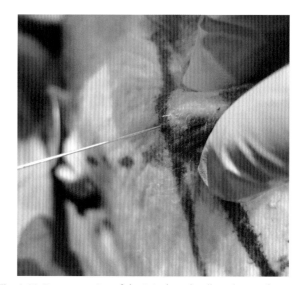

Fig. 1.11 Demonstration of the "pinch-and-pull" technique for penetration of a blunt cannula into a suborbicularis plane into the prezygomatic space. (From Surek C, Beut J, Stephens R, Lamb J, Jelks G. Volumizing viaducts of the midface: defining the Beut techniques. Aesthet Surg J 2015;35(2):121–134 with permission)

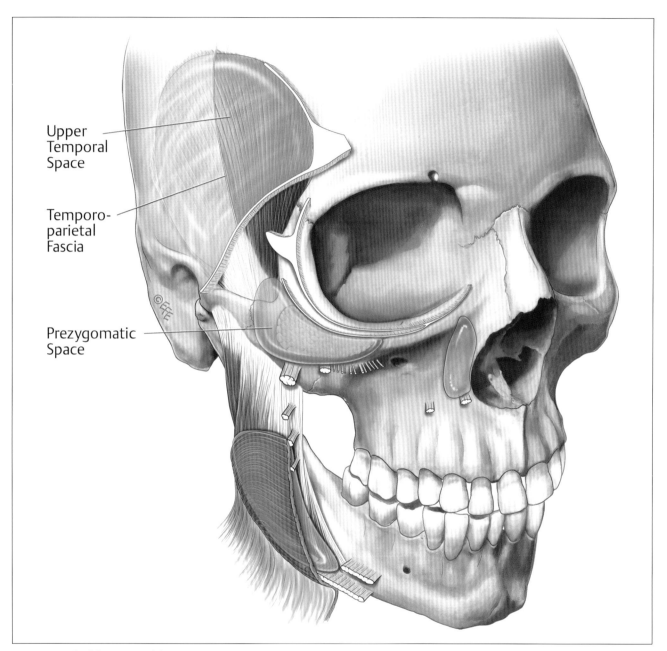

Upper
Temporal
Space

Temporo-
parietal
Fascia

Prezygomatic
Space

Fig. 1.12 Medical illustration of the prezygomatic space.

The Medial and Lateral Suborbicularis Oculi Fat Compartments and the Deep Medial Cheek Fat Compartment

The Upper Midface

The SOOF is a thin layer of fat residing between the undersurface of the orbicularis oculi muscle and the dense posterior capsule of SMAS. The SOOF is partitioned into medial and lateral components by an arterial branch supplying the palpebral eyelid.

The Lower Midface

The unique anatomical architecture of the lower midface exists caudal to the zygomaticocutaneous ligaments. The deep medial cheek fat (DMCF) compartment has been found to become deficient in volume with age and is associated with small adipocyte size, in contrast to the supra-SMAS fat compartments that have been shown to hypertrophy with age. Initially described by Pessa and Rohrich in cadaveric dissection, the three-dimensional construct of the DMCF was studied through computed tomography by Mathias Gierloff.

By definition, the deep medial cheek compartment lies anterior to the zygomaticomaxillary buttress. The DMCF is partitioned by the levator anguli oris creating medal and lateral components.

The Lateral Component of the Deep Medial Cheek Fat

The ill-defined lateral border of this DMCF abuts the buccal space and bony maxillary depression. In cadaveric study, the lateral component of the DMCF has demonstrated a loose, areolar consistency. The authors do not recommend the lateral component as a target for deep cheek volumization.

The Medial Component of the Deep Medial Cheek Fat

The medial component of the DMCF is wedged between the premaxillary space anteriorly and deep pyriform space posteriorly. This fat is more robust and compact compared to its lateral counterpart. Volumization of the medial DMCF along with the deep pyriform space has been postulated to enhance anterior cheek projection in the aging face and may create a fulcrum effect on the draping lip elevators that traverse superficial to the compartment. For topographic identification, the medial component of the DMCF lies within an area less than 1.5 cm lateral to the base of the alar crease (**Figs. 1.13**, **1.14**).

Injection Pearl

Inject deep and medial in the anterior cheek. Choose filler composition wisely. We recommend medium to large particle size filler with high cohesivity or autologous fat.

Fig. 1.15 shows the gross anatomy of the fat compartments discussed in this section.

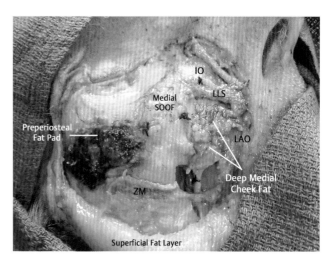

Fig. 1.13 Lateral view. The superficial fat compartments have been retracted. Zygomaticus major (ZM) and levator labii superioris (LLS) are labeled. The orbicularis oculi has been resected. Remnants of the lateral suborbicularis oculi fat compartment (SOOF) are noted on top of the preperiosteal fat (PPF). The medial SOOF and the infraorbital (IO) neurovascular bundle are labeled. The loose areolar consistency of the deep medial cheek fat is noted lateral to the transected levator anguli oris (LAO). (From Surek CC, Beut J, Stephens R, Jelks G, Lamb J. Pertinent anatomy and analysis for midface volumizing procedures. Plast Reconstr Surg 2015;135(5):818e–829e with permission)

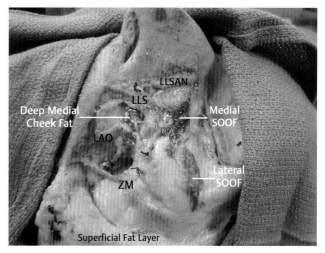

Fig. 1.14 Lateral view. The superficial fat compartment layer has been reflected. The orbicularis oculi has been resected. Demonstration of the deep medial cheek fat (DMCF) and medial suborbicularis oculi fat compartment (SOOF) stained with methylene blue. The zygomaticus major (ZM), levator anguli oris (LAO), levator labii superioris (LLS), and levator labii superioris alaeque nasi (LLSAN) are labeled. Hyaluronic acid filler homogenized with red dye has been injected into the lateral SOOF overlying the preperiosteal fat compartment. (From Surek CC, Beut J, Stephens R, Jelks G, Lamb J. Pertinent anatomy and analysis for midface volumizing procedures. Plast Reconstr Surg 2015;135(5):818e–829e with permission)

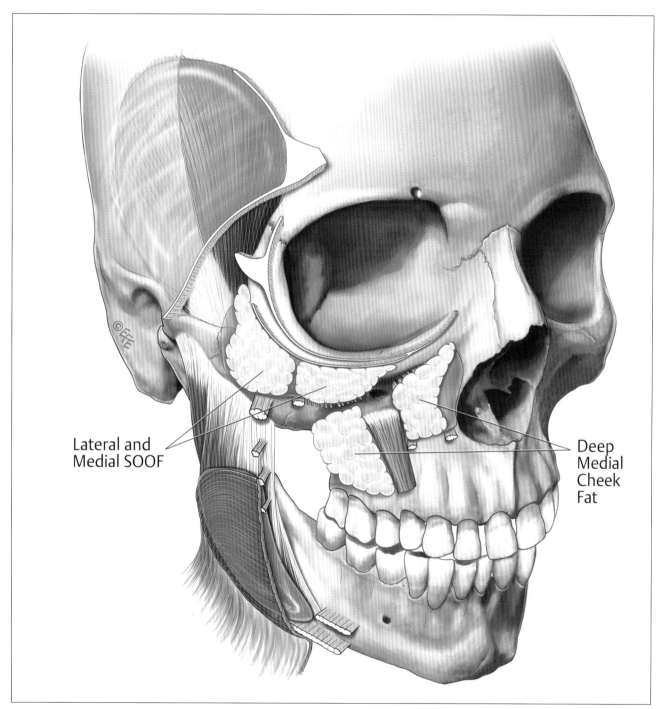

Fig. 1.15 Medical illustration of the sub-SMAS (subsuperficial muscular aponeurotic system) fat compartments in the midface.

The Facial Nerve

The facial nerve exits the stylomastoid foramen and divides into five main branches:

- The frontal or temporal branch.
- The zygomatic branch.
- The buccal branch.
- The marginal mandibular branch.
- The cervical branch.

The Frontal or Temporal Branch

Traditional teaching relates the path of this nerve to a topographic "Pitanguy" line beginning 0.5 cm inferior to the tragus and coursing to a point 1.5 cm lateral to the supraorbital rim. Anatomically, the nerve remains deep to SMAS until it transcends superficial along the undersurface of the temporoparietal fascia approximately 2 cm above the zygomatic arch. The nerve does have an intimate relationship with the anterior branch of the superficial temporal artery. When the nerve reaches the level of the sentinel vein, it resides superficial to the vein in the roof of the lower temporal space.

The Zygomatic Branch

The zygomatic branch traverses within the parotid gland; as it exits anteriorly, it lies caudal to the zygoma and cephalic to the parotid duct. It continues along the masseter muscle coursing with the transverse facial artery. At the main zygomatic liga-ment, this nerve provides a branch to the lower orbicularis oculi muscle. The nerve then continues medially and innervates the undersurface of the zygomaticus major and minor muscles.

The Buccal Branch

The upper and lower buccal trunks travel within the masseter fascia. Upon reaching the anterior border of the masseter, these nerves traverse superficially alongside the upper and lower masseteric ligaments, respectively.

The Marginal Mandibular Branch

At the angle of the mandible, this nerve courses within the platysma-auricular fascia and continues anteriorly along the masseter toward the level of the mandibular ligament. Traditional teaching states that 81% of branches travel superior to the mandibular border and that all branches are superior to the mandibular once the nerve traverses anterior to the facial artery and vein.

The Cervical Branch

This nerve usually contains a series of branches that course inferiorly into the neck to supply platysma muscle fibers.

Fig. 1.16 presents the gross anatomy of the five main branches of the facial nerve.

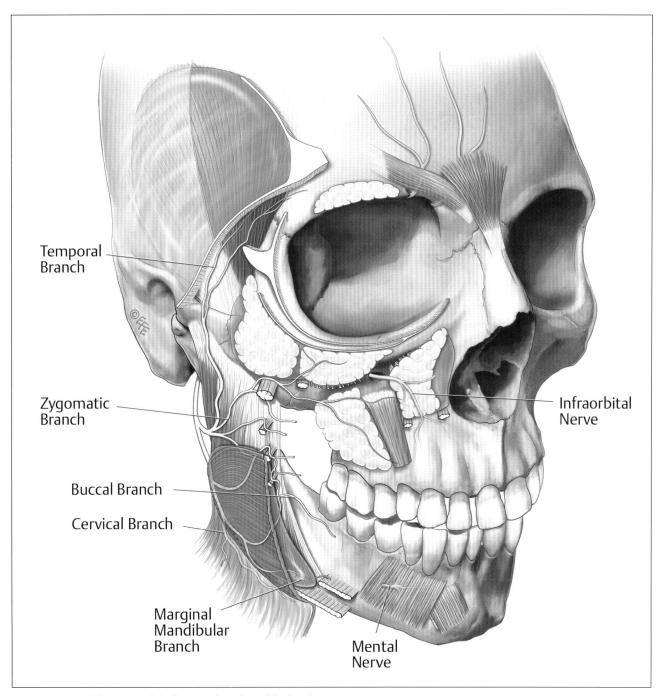

Temporal
Branch

Zygomatic
Branch

Buccal Branch

Cervical Branch

Infraorbital
Nerve

Marginal
Mandibular
Branch

Mental
Nerve

Fig. 1.16 Medical illustration of the five main branches of the facial nerve.

The Vascular Anatomy of the Midface

Arterial Anatomy of the Midface

We will address perioral vascular anatomy in the next chapter. In regard to the midface, we begin with the angular artery (**Video 1.3**). The topographic approximation of the angular artery origin is the intersection of a horizontal line from the supratip break of the nose and a vertical midpupillary line, roughly 3.5 cm from the midline. Traditionally the angular artery will traverse cephalic to the medial commissure of the alar–facial groove joining the dorsal nasal branch of the ophthalmic artery. A detoured course of the angular artery has been observed up to 30%; this artery takes a more lateral trajectory near the nasojugal groove coursing along the inferior border of the orbicularis oculi toward the facial midsagittal line. Knowledge of this anatomic variation is important for injectors filling the nasojugal groove. In the inferior palpebral and infraorbital regions of the face, these artery branches emerge into the subcutaneous layer, making them potentially vulnerable during tear trough and nasojugal groove injections. These findings give credence to cannula injections in the deep suborbicularis plane for effacement of these aging phenomena.

Pessa and Rohrich describe the junction of the lid-cheek crease and nasojugal crease as a suitable topographic landmark to identify the emergence of the infraorbital neurovascular bundle. An ascending branch of the infraorbital artery traverses over the preperiosteal fat. This has been previously described as the palpebral branch of the infraorbital artery (PIOA). In cadaver studies, this bundle has been identified traversing the medial SOOF compartment as it ascends to the palpebral fissure.

Hwang et al reported the location of PIOA to be approximately half the eye width from the medial canthus. The angular artery location can be topographically approximated by a point 1.7 mm from the midline and 1.3 cm inferior to the medial canthus.

Venous Anatomy of the Midface

The angular vein is untethered from deeper structures by the presence of sub-SMAS anatomic spaces as it courses in the lateral boundary of the premaxillary space. Medial and cephalic to the bounds of these spaces, the angular vein has significant reduced mobility, and becomes intimate with preperiosteal tissues as it nears the medial canthus and tears trough ligament origin. The angular vein, which is anterior to the medial canthal tendon on the lateral side of the nose, curves along the inferomedial boundary of the orbicularis oculi. Once the vein is at least 5 mm lateral to the medial canthus, it freely floats with the orbicularis oculi muscle edge and its posterior capsule. Cadaver dissection has revealed a tethering of the angular vein at the level of the tear trough ligament. The authors believe this explains the engorgement of the vein following superficial tear trough volumizing procedures. This can create a significant prominence of that vein over the lateral upper nasal wall and lacrimal region.

Injection Pearl

The injector must have a keen understanding of the DEPTH of all structures in the upper midface to avoid unwanted outcomes.

Fig. 1.17 depicts the gross vascular anatomy of the midface.

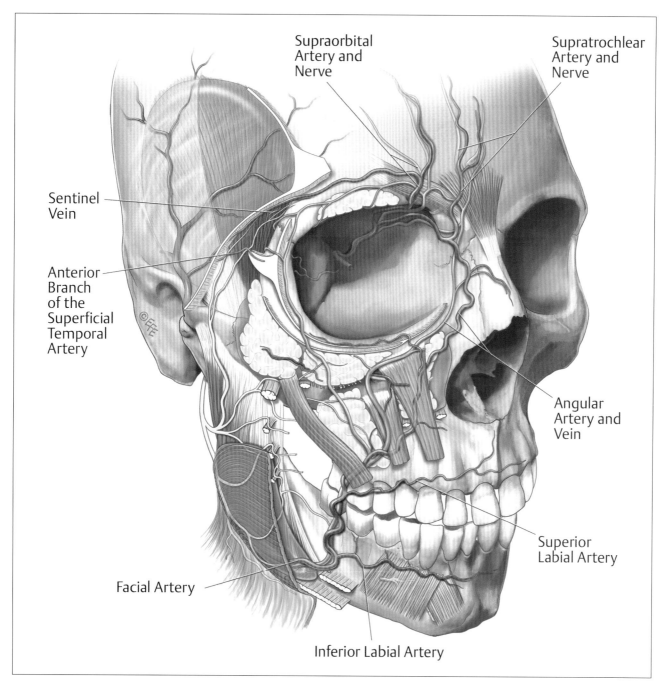

Supraorbital Artery and Nerve

Supratrochlear Artery and Nerve

Sentinel Vein

Anterior Branch of the Superficial Temporal Artery

Angular Artery and Vein

Superior Labial Artery

Facial Artery

Inferior Labial Artery

Fig. 1.17 Medical illustration of the high-yield venous and arterial anatomy of the face.

The Premaxillary Space

Superficial to the deep medial cheek compartment lies the SMAS. The SMAS is robust on the undersurface of the superficial medial cheek fat compartment, but becomes attenuated as it nears the nasolabial crease. On the anterior surface of the medial component of the deep medial cheek compartment lies the levator labii superioris (LLS) and subsequent premaxillary space. This space extends beneath the posterior capsule of the orbicularis oculi muscle, which is contiguous with SMAS. The infraorbital neurovascular bundle lies on the floor of this space on the anterior surface of the LLS. The angular vein traverses on the lateral border of the space.

Clinically, the injector can access both the premaxillary space and the deep pyriform space with blunt cannulas. Once the cannula penetrates the skin and traverses subcutaneous, the angle of cannula vector facilitates the injector's ability to determine which space the cannula resides. Anatomically, once the cannula is deep to the nasolabial fold, the cannula has reached a sub-SMAS plane. A shallow 30-degree vector will place the cannula in the premaxillary space. A steeper, 60- to 90-degree, vector down to bone will safely place the cannula within the deep pyriform space (**Figs. 1.18**, **1.19**).

The clinical confirmation that the cannula has arrived in either of the targeted spaces is a perceptible free passage and movement of the cannula. If the injector feels resistance, the cannula is likely in the DMCF. Anecdotally, we recommend highly cohesive filler, hydroxyapatite, or autologous fat for deep pyriform space volumization. We do not recommend aqueous-based filler for volumization of these spaces.

The gross anatomy of the premaxillary space is shown in **Fig. 1.20**.

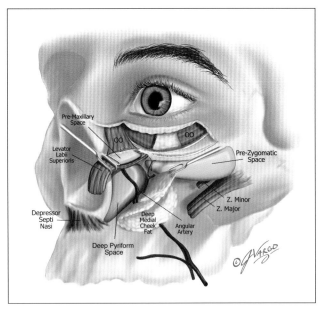

Fig. 1.18 Medical illustration of the deep pyriform space and important adjacent anatomical structures.

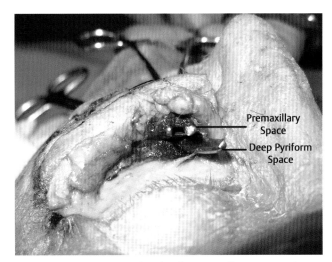

Fig. 1.19 Instruments are placed in the premaxillary space and the deep pyriform. The instruments were advanced through the tear trough ligament demonstrating that these structures reside in distinctly different planes. (From Surek C, Vargo J, Lamb J. Deep pyriform space: anatomical clarifications and clinical implications. Plast Reconstr Surg. 2016;138(1). 2016 with permission)

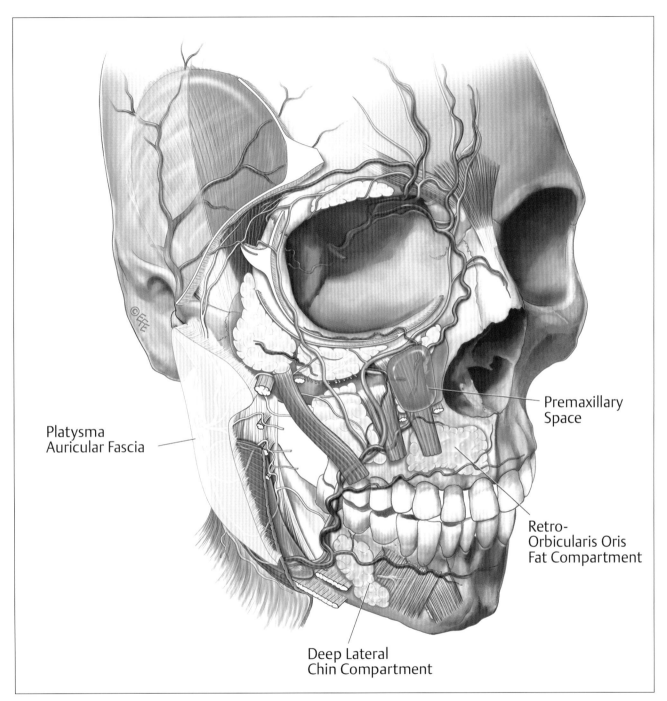

Platysma
Auricular Fascia

Premaxillary
Space

Retro-
Orbicularis Oris
Fat Compartment

Deep Lateral
Chin Compartment

Fig. 1.20 Medical illustration of the premaxillary space and the platysma-auricular fascia.

The Infraorbital Fat Compartment "Malar Bag" and the Superficial Cheek Compartments

The Upper Midface

Superficial to the orbicularis oculi muscle lies the malar fat compartment, which is also synonymous with the infraorbital fat compartment. The orbicularis oculi muscle and the malar fat compartment anatomically stain as a solitary tissue space drained by a single lymphatic channel that drains into a buccal node (**Fig. 1.21**). Caution should be exercised if injecting this space, as diminished lymphatics may lead to a persistent periorbital edema and iatrogenic malar bags (**Fig. 1.22**).

Upper Midface Pitfall 1

Iatrogenic malar mound: "The bee sting appearance."
Explanation: Superficial injection into the infraorbital fat pad.

Anatomically, the malar bag is formed between the cutaneous insertions of the ORL and the zygomaticocutaneous ligaments. Authors refer to the cutaneous insertion of the ORL as the palpebromalar groove. This groove is the lateral continuation of the tear trough. The malar bag is not to be confused with a festoon, which by definition is hypertrophy of the orbicularis oculi muscle. Guy Massry has described the malar mound as either a wet or a dry festoon. Likely, the wet festoon represents a lymphatic dysfunction, whereas the dry festoon represents a cutaneous laxity/excess.

The superficial lateral, middle, medial, and nasolabial fat compartments are bounded by vascularized septae. Adipocyte size in these spaces increases with rising BMI (body mass index). The conjecture that deep fat compartments are less responsive to lipid metabolism and weight changes is controversial. It has been postulated that aging volume loss begins in the lateral superficial compartment and transitions medially. This has been correlated to progression and severity of the submalar hollow and nasojugal groove with facial aging. In essence, these topographic changes can act as an anecdotal scale to grade the degree of facial aging in patients.

Volume within these compartments may support and give turgor to the cutaneous structures and gauge the distribution of tension within the collagenous subdermal fibers described as Langer's lines. Though not always appreciated, the Langer's lines of skin in the immediate subdermal tissues are relevant to how volumizing procedures determine resultant cheek shape. Expansion of the superficial spaces can affect cheek convexity through superolateral displacement of those parallel bundles. During cannula-based procedures, the bounds of the superficial medial and middle compartments are readily apparent as resistance is felt when passing the cannula through the vascularized septa that divide them. Gierloff has described a superficial extension of the deep buccal fat pad that can provide support to the caudal boundary of both these superficial spaces.

Injection Pearl

Grooves and surface creases are associated with superficial lymphatics; filling these grooves can block lymphatics and distort animation.

Injection Pearl

When injecting superficial fat, inject PERPENDICULAR to Langer's lines.

Fig. 1.23 shows the gross anatomy of the fat compartments discussed in this section.

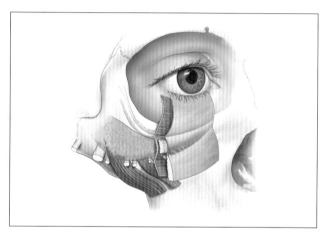

Fig. 1.21 Illustration of the anatomical depth relationships in the upper midface. The prezygomatic space is demonstrated in the deep suborbicularis plane (blue capsule). The orbitomalar ligament is demonstrated arborizing through the orbicularis oculi muscle inserting into the skin forming the tear trough crease. The zygomaticocutaneous ligaments arborize through the orbicularis forming a partition between the infraorbital "malar" fat compartment superiorly and superficial cheek compartment inferiorly. The cutaneous insertion of the ligaments forms the characteristic skin crease demonstrated in clinical malar mounds.

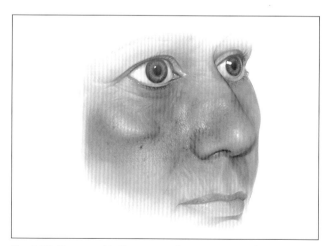

Fig. 1.22 Photographic illustration of an iatrogenic malar mound resulting from superficial injection in the infraorbital "malar" fat compartment. Note the cutaneous insertions of the orbitomalar ligament superiorly and the zygomaticocutaneous ligaments inferiorly.

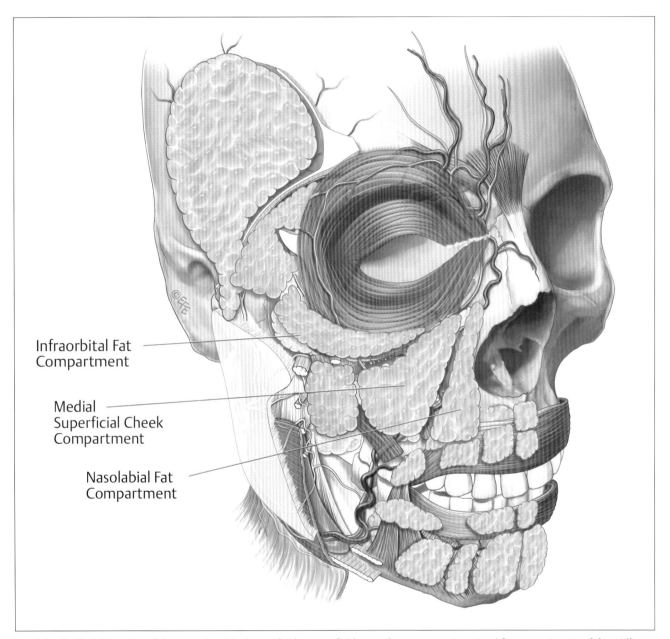

Infraorbital Fat
Compartment

Medial
Superficial Cheek
Compartment

Nasolabial Fat
Compartment

Fig. 1.23 Medical illustration of the supra-SMAS (subsuperficial to superficial muscularo-aponeurotic system) fat compartments of the midface.

The Authors' Preferred Techniques for Midfacial Volumization

Deep Volumization

Midface volume addition techniques are first divided into features of aging addressing tissue dissent/sagging versus skeletal deficiencies. The goal is optimized volume rejuvenation in the areas of most notable deficiency. A compartment and sub-SMAS space-based approach using medium to high-G prime filler or autologous fat augmentation is targeted at areas of diminished ligamentous and soft-tissue support.

Lateral Midface (Deep Injection)

Individuals showing a significant nasojugal fold will likely be deficient in several areas. First an assessment is made of lower eyelid vector. In individuals with a negative vector, the primary augmentation site will be the prezygomatic space (**Video 1.2**). An injection port 1.5 cm inferolateral to the lateral canthus is utilized. A pinch-and-pull technique with the noninjection hand facilitates cannula passage through the prezygomatic space capsule. This capsule is analogous to the investment of

SMAS on the posterior surface of the orbicularis oculi muscle. A palpable and often audible "pop" is noted when the cannula penetrates this capsule. Once in the prezygomatic space, the injector can move the cannula freely along the upper maxilla. The prezygomatic space has roughly the shape of a Silastic cheek implant. The space extends superolateral up to the point of the lateral orbital thickening, which is the extension of the lateral canthal structures. The injector can sweep the cannula within the space to feel the caudal boundary (zygomaticocutaneous ligaments) and the cephalic boundary (ORL). Volume additions of approximately 0.6 mL with off-the-shelf fillers or fat grafting volumes of approximately 1.4 to 1.5 mL are typical in this space.

Anterior Midface (Deep Injection)

The authors' preferred technique for effacement of tear troughs is vertical cannula injections of autologous fat or off-the-shelf HA (hyaluronic acid) fillers placed in a vertical stalagmite fashion via the deep pyriform or premaxillary spaces (**Video 1.4**). These are accessed through a port roughly 1.5 cm inferolateral from the alar base in the nasolabial crease.

Fig. 1.24 illustrates the authors' preferred technique for deep volumization of the midface.

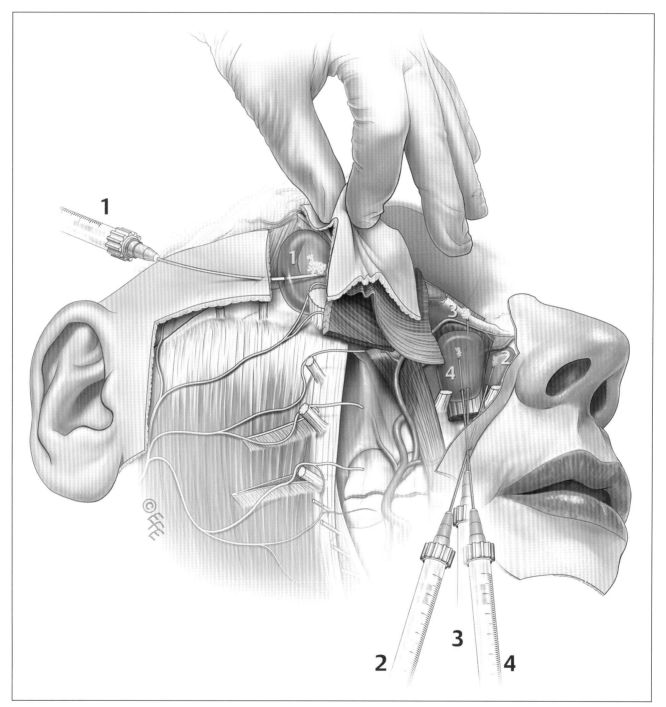

Fig. 1.24 Medical illustration depicting the authors' preferred technique for deep volumization in the anterior and lateral midface.

Superficial Volumization

Lateral Midface (Superficial Injection)

Due to the lateral limitation of the prezygomatic space, volumization in the space does not address the lateral zygoma sweep. To address this, the injector can perform the DeMaio V1 injection (**Video 1.5**), which overlies the zygomaticotemporal suture. A bolus injection in this location of approximately 0.25 to 0.4 mL will have a transmitted effect across the convexity of the cheek. Additionally, the DeMaio V2 injection is placed on the cephalic border of the main zygomatic ligament and should further enhance lateral cheek projection.

Anterior Midface (Superficial Injection)

Loss of turgor within the cheek along with overall decrease in cheek radius is addressed with superficial filler injections or fat grafting in the supra-SMAS fat compartments. The primary targets are the superficial middle and medial fat compartments as described by Pessa et al. These are accessed through a port roughly 1.5 cm inferolateral from the alar base in the nasolabial crease. The bounds of the superficial medial and middle compartments are readily apparent as resistance is felt when passing the cannula through the vascularized septae that divide them (**Fig. 1.25**). The injector can fan broadly across these compartments to blend them, restoring volume and contour.

When a contour step-off is evident between the curvature of the cheek and the inferior aspect of the lateral fat pad of the eyelid, an injection as espoused by Arthur Swift is beneficial. This injection is targeted cephalic to the anticipated course of the zygomaticofacial bundle. It is recommended that a reflux maneuver is performed with this injection to ensure the injection does not enter a vessel. Generally, for this injection, HA fillers are blended with additional Xylocaine. Due to this increase in volume, the needle is lifted slightly to tent the tissues prior to injection and after reflux. This injection is performed with sharp needle and the authors do not recommend cannula injection of fat in this location.

Fig. 1.26 demonstrates the authors' preferred technique for superficial volumization of the midface.

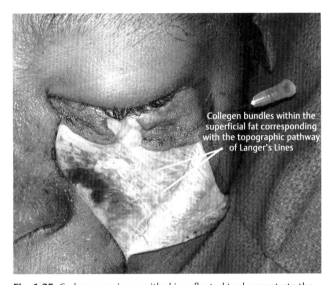

Collegen bundles within the superficial fat corresponding with the topographic pathway of Langer's Lines

Fig. 1.25 Cadaver specimen with skin reflected to demonstrate the collagen elastin bundles in the superficial fat corresponding to the pathway of Langer's lines.

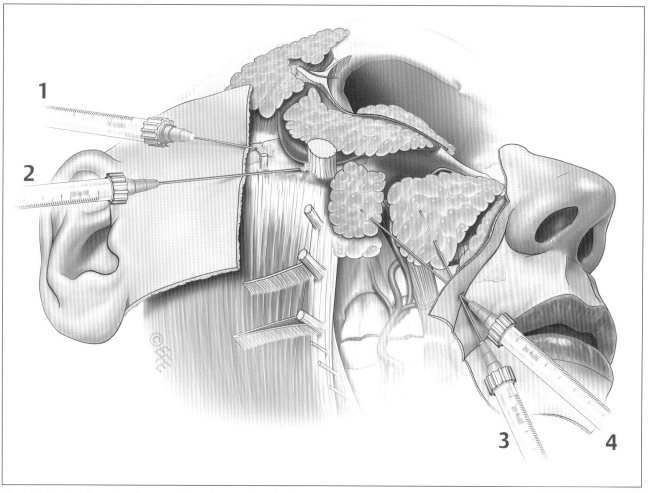

Fig. 1.26 Medical illustration depicting the authors' preferred technique for superficial volumization in the anterior and lateral midface with deep bolus injections per DeMaio.

Suggested Reading

Aiache AE, Ramirez OH. The suborbicularis oculi fat pads: an anatomic and clinical study. Plast Reconstr Surg 1995;95(1):37–42

Alghoul M, Codner MA. Retaining ligaments of the face: review of anatomy and clinical applications. Aesthet Surg J 2013;33(6):769–782

Cotofana S, Schenck TL, Trevidic P, et al. Midface: clinical anatomy and regional approaches with injectable fillers. Plast Reconstr Surg 2015; 136(5, Suppl):219S–234S

Donofrio LM. Fat distribution: a morphologic study of the aging face. Dermatol Surg 2000;26(12):1107–1112

Faras J, Pessa J, Hubbard B, et al. The science and theory behind facial aging. Plastic and Reconstructive Surgery –Global Open 2013; 1(1):e8–e15

Furnas DW. The retaining ligaments of the cheek. Plast Reconstr Surg 1989;83(1):11–16

Gierloff M, Stöhring C, Buder T, Wiltfang J. The subcutaneous fat compartments in relation to aesthetically important facial folds and rhytides. J Plast Reconstr Aesthet Surg 2012;65(10):1292–1297

Gierloff M, Stöhring C, Buder T, Gassling V, Açil Y, Wiltfang J. Aging changes of the midfacial fat compartments: a computed tomographic study. Plast Reconstr Surg 2012;129(1):263–273

Gosain AK, Klein MH, Sudhakar PV, Prost RW. A volumetric analysis of soft-tissue changes in the aging midface using high-resolution MRI: implications for facial rejuvenation. Plast Reconstr Surg 2005;115(4):1143–1152, discussion 1153–1155

Guyuron B, Rowe DJ, Weinfeld AB, Eshraghi Y, Fathi A, Iamphongsai S. Factors contributing to the facial aging of identical twins. Plast Reconstr Surg 2009;123(4):1321–1331

Kikkawa DO, Lemke BN, Dortzbach RK. Relations of the superficial musculoaponeurotic system to the orbit and characterization of the orbitomalar ligament. Ophthal Plast Reconstr Surg 1996;12(2):77–88

Lambros V. Observations on periorbital and midface aging. Plast Reconstr Surg 2007;120(5):1367–1376, discussion 1377

Mendelson B, Wong C. Anatomy of the aging face. In: Neligan PC, ed. Plastic Surgery. Vol. 2. 3rd ed. Philadelphia, PA: Elsevier Saunders; 2013:78–92

Pessa J, Rohrich R. Facial Topography: Clinical Anatomy of the Face. St. Louis, MO: Quality Medical Publishing; 2012

Stuzin JM, Baker TJ, Gordon HL. The relationship of the superficial and deep facial fascias: relevance to rhytidectomy and aging. Plast Reconstr Surg 1992;89(3):441–449, discussion 450–451

Surek CC, Beut J, Stephens R, Jelks G, Lamb J. Pertinent anatomy and analysis for midface volumizing procedures. Plast Reconstr Surg 2015;135(5):818e–829e

Surek C, Beut J, Stephens R, Lamb J, Jelks G. Volumizing viaducts of the midface: defining the Beut techniques. Aesthet Surg J 2015;35(2):121–134

Wan D, Amirlak B, Giessler P, et al. The differing adipocyte morphologies of deep versus superficial midfacial fat compartments: a cadaveric study. Plast Reconstr Surg 2014;133(5):615e–622e

Wan D, Amirlak B, Rohrich R, Davis K. The clinical importance of the fat compartments in midfacial aging. Plast Reconstr Surg Glob Open 2014; 1–8

Wong CH, Mendelson B. Facial soft-tissue spaces and retaining ligaments of the midcheek: defining the premaxillary space. Plast Reconstr Surg 2013;132(1):49–56

Wong CH, Hsieh MK, Mendelson B. The tear trough ligament: anatomical basis for the tear trough deformity. Plast Reconstr Surg 2012;129(6):1392–1402

Yang HM, Lee JG, Hu KS, et al. New anatomical insights on the course and branching patterns of the facial artery: clinical implications of injectable treatments to the nasolabial fold and nasojugal groove. Plast Reconstr Surg 2014;133(5):1077–1082

Chapter 2

**The Lymphatic Anatomy
of the Lower Eyelid
and the Malar Region
of the Face**

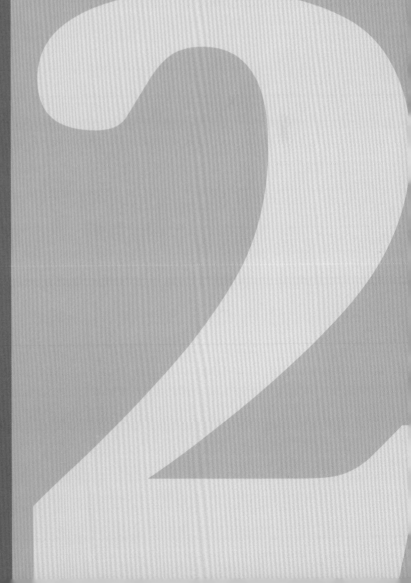

2 The Lymphatic Anatomy of the Lower Eyelid and the Malar Region of the Face

Sajna Shoukath and Mark Winter Ashton

A keen understanding of facial lymphatics is the missing link in the anatomy of facial injections. This knowledge equips the injector with a secret weapon in their armamentarium to prevent suboptimal aesthetic outcomes secondary to prolonged lymphedema. In particular, this emphasizes the importance of injection depth in the midface.

We would like to thank Dr. Shoukath and Professor Ashton for their fantastic work on facial lymphatics, a series of findings relevant to the injector and fat grafting surgeon. Iatrogenic persistent periorbital edema may be the result of lymphatic injury, lymphatic fouling, or possibly particle cohesivity in the case of hyaluronic acid fillers. Cannula techniques for volume placement in the prezygomatic space, when entered laterally in a mobile segment of the periorbital, should provide safety as the cannula is directed toward malar periosteum and then advanced medially. Sharp needle injection in the region of the bilamellar orbital retaining ligament poses some risk of injury or impingement of the deep lateral lymphatic channel. Based upon anatomic dissections in the region of the zygomaticomaxillary retaining ligament, the caudal border of the prezygomatic space is a series of osteocutaneous ligaments, rather than a membranous structure as is present cephalad in the orbital retaining ligament. As such, volume-based procedures near the caudal aspect of the prezygomatic space would theoretically be less prone to an impingement since the lymphatics do not pierce a dense anatomic structure.

—Jerome P. Lamb and Christopher C. Surek

Introduction

Our knowledge of the human lymphatic system is predominantly based on the pioneering work of Sappey[1] and his successors[2] in the 19th and early 20th centuries. This is because the lymphatic system is extremely difficult to study; the vessels are small and fragile, and the presence of multiple valves makes retrograde filling of the lymphatic system for radiographic analysis impossible.

Recent advances in the imaging of the lymphatic system, particularly the use of hydrogen peroxide, have allowed for new studies of lymphatic architecture that were previously not possible.[3] This is important because many of the questions concerning lymphatic anatomy are not answered by the existing literature.[4]

Analogous to the venous system, the lymphatic system of the human body is initially composed of a very fine capillary network, the vessels of which measure only 20 to 70 μm in diameter.[5] This network subsequently drains into larger "precollecting" vessels (70–150 μm) located in the deep dermis. Both the "capillaries" and "precollectors" are avalvular. From here, lymph is directed more deeply into lymph "collecting" vessels. These are larger, measuring 150 to 350 μm, and most importantly contain multiple valves that serve to direct lymph to a predetermined, singular and specific "sentinel" lymph node.[6]

Facial Lymphatics

Within the face, lymphatic fluid is primarily directed to the parotid and submandibular lymph nodes.[7] It does so via a superficial and deep series of collecting vessels that are consistent and predictable in their location. Knowledge of the location of these collecting vessels is critical in facial revolumization procedures as the fragile and compressible nature of the collecting lymphatic vessels means that they can be easily occluded, leading to subsequent lymphedema in the tissue they drain (**Fig. 2.1**).

The lower eyelid and its conjunctiva is particularly susceptible to lymphedema and chemosis. Indeed, the recent trend to more aggressive surgery around the lateral extent of the orbital retaining ligament (ORL) has been accompanied by an increase in postoperative periorbital chemosis. As an example, published complication rates of persistent chemosis beyond 2 to 3 weeks have risen from a traditional low rate of 0.8 to 1%[8] to up to 34.5% in one series recently published.[9] In each published series, the increased chemosis rate was accompanied by more aggressive surgery in the lower eyelid, the ORL, and the malar complex.

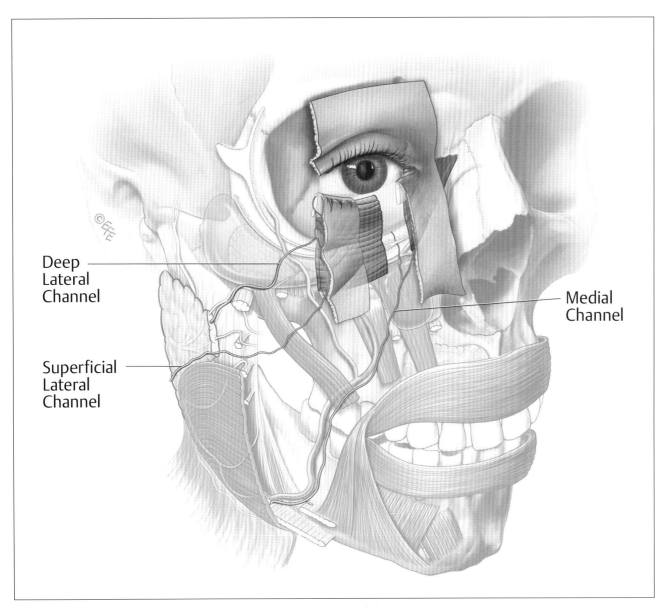

Deep
Lateral
Channel

Superficial
Lateral
Channel

Medial
Channel

Fig. 2.1 Illustration of the lymphatic channels of the midface and the lower eyelid.

We know that arteries, nerves, and veins cross tissue planes at points of ligamentous fixation. We also know that the face can be divided into five distinct tissue layers (**Fig. 2.2**) and that the location of nerves and arteries within these planes is consistent.[10] Elsewhere in the body, the precollecting lymphatic vessels are located in the deepest subsection of layer 2, called 2C.[5] The main collecting trunks travel in layer 4.[5] The face is no different. The capillary network within the conjunctiva of the lower eyelid and eye drains into precollectors in the deep dermis of the conjunctiva and travels superficial to the preseptal orbicularis oculi muscle in the same layer (2C). Broadly, these precollectors fall into two groups: those orientated toward the medial canthus (the medial system) and those directed toward the lateral canthus (the lateral system).

At the medial third of the ORL, the medial system of precollectors coalesces to form a collecting trunk, which turns inferiorly, and travelling within a discrete fat compartment, continues within the nasolabial fat compartment[11] to drain into the submandibular lymph node. The lateral group of precollectors coalesce at the lateral third of the ORL and turn inferolaterally within the lateral orbital fat compartment[11] to drain into the preauricular lymph nodes.[12] These two medial and lateral systems comprise the superficial lymphatic system.

As would be predicted, there is an additional system of lymphatic vessels running deep to the orbicularis oculi muscle, that is, in layer 4. This deep system drains the lower eyelid and upper mid cheek directly from precollectors traveling through the tarsal plate and Meibomian glands in the lateral third of the lower eyelid. This deep lymphatic system is joined by connections with the superficial lymphatic system by precollectors that travel directly through the preseptal orbicularis muscle to link the superficial system in layer 2 with the deep system in layer 4.

Lymphatic precollectors of the deep system travel beneath the preseptal orbicularis. Laterally, in the lateral lower quadrant at the junction of the ORL and the lateral orbital thickening (LOT), the precollectors pass through the superficial ORL and coalesce to form larger collecting lymphatics that travel in the suborbicularis oculi fat (SOOF) within the roof of the prezygomatic space. At the level of the most cranial zygomaticocutaneous ligaments (ZCL), that is, at the point of fixation, the collectors vertically descend into the preperiosteal fat surrounding the origin of zygomaticus major (ZM). There, the lateral deep collectors descend beneath the deep fascia to travel with the facial nerve to reach the preauricular lymph nodes within the parotid.

An equivalent medial deep facial lymphatic system has not been identified despite extensive searching. Given histological evidence of deep lymphatic vessels in the medial eyelid, it is probable that this system also exists but may be smaller or less developed than the lateral system.

Thus, there are three main lymphatic channels of the lower eyelid and mid cheek. Lymphatic channels within the medial lower eyelid coalesce to form a superficial medial system, while the lymphatics of the lateral eyelid form both a superficial and a deep lateral system of lymphatics. The medial system drains to the submandibular gland, and the lateral system drains to the parotid.

As would be predicted from elsewhere in the body, the capillary network and the precollectors located within the conjunctiva are avalvular and there is free communication between the medial and lateral eye. There is also a free communication between precollectors of the lower and upper eyelids around the lateral canthus. Our studies would suggest that the majority of lymphatic drainage from both the upper and lower eyelids is through the lateral system.[6,7]

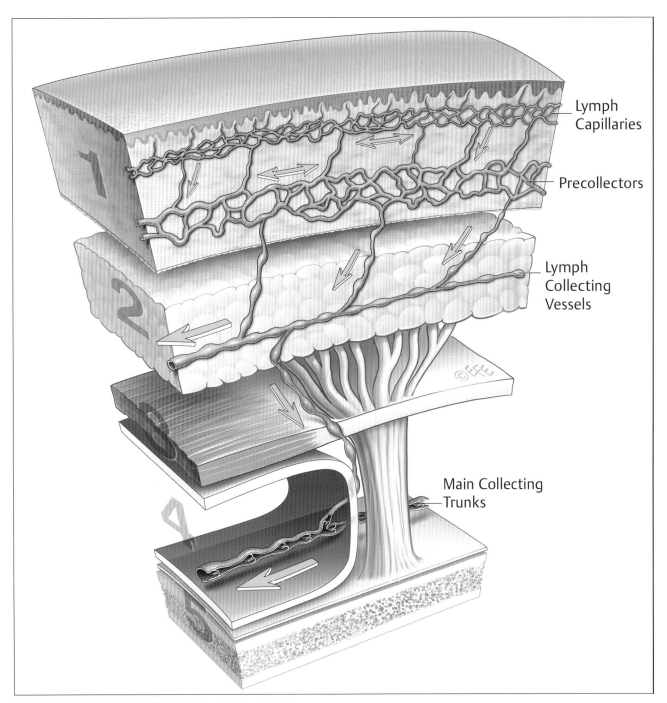

Fig. 2.2 Illustration of the facial lymphatic architecture.

Ramifications for the Surgeon

Prolonged malar and lid swelling was first noted by Hamra[13] in his composite rhytidectomy technique in which much of the dissection was in the plane over orbicularis oculi at the junction with subcutaneous fat. A study utilizing lymphoscintigraphy has suggested that such extensive dissection during a rhytidectomy may cause increased edema postoperatively by decreasing lymphatic outflow.[14] Increased rates of lower eyelid edema have been described[15] as incisions for orbital fracture fixation became more caudal on the face. Mendelson et al[16] noted that excision of subcutaneous fat in malar mounds lead to prolonged swelling.

New studies into lymphatic anatomy of the lower eyelid and malar region have provided an insight into the anatomic basis for these observations.[12] The collecting vessels of the superficial lymphatic system are formed superficial to the preseptal orbicularis muscle approximately 10 mm from the lid margin in precisely the region of the infraorbital incisions described earlier. These vessels also travel within previously described subcutaneous fat compartments.[11] Previous studies have reported that lymphatic collector vessels take approximately 3 weeks to be reformed after injury,[17] and hence, it can be expected that damage to these vessels will lead to prolonged lower eyelid and cheek edema while they are being repaired.

Further, it is now that clear that lymphatic vessels draining the conjunctiva do so via an additional deep network of lymphatics in which the lymphatic capillaries of the conjunctiva are also able to drain into the deep system via precollectors traveling through the tarsal plate laterally. The deep lymphatic collectors subsequently formed are deep to the preseptal orbicularis oculi and are located at the junction of the orbicularis retaining ligament's junction with the LOT. These collecting vessels then course through the superficial portion of the ORL to travel in the SOOF in the roof of the prezygomatic space. At the most cranial ZCL,[10] the collectors descend to the preperiosteal fat around the ZM origin and then travel beneath the deep fascia adjacent to the facial nerve to drain into preauricular lymph nodes within the parotid.

By scrutinizing the reported chemosis rates in various lower eyelid blepharoplasty techniques (**Table 2.1**), it becomes clear that the incidence of chemosis increases as the dissection in the procedure becomes deeper and more lateral. Skin–muscle flap lower eyelid blepharoplasty has a reported chemosis rate of 1%,[8] attributable to the minimal amount of dissection around the lateral canthus and the orbicularis retaining ligament. Transconjunctival access has rates of chemosis ranging from 0.8 to 7.6%,[18,19] even when combined with deep dissection around the ORL, presumably because the superficial lymphatic network is not injured. It is notable that in both of these techniques, only one of the lymphatic systems of the face is potentially damaged. As the superficial and deep lymphatic systems of the face have interconnections through the preseptal orbicularis, it is probable that damage to one system will be compensated for by the other without chemosis occurring.

However, when both the deep and the superficial systems are damaged, lymphatic outflow of the lower eyelid is severely compromised and relies on cross-connections with a potentially less developed medial drainage system. It is therefore proposed that damage to the deep system, in addition to the superficial system, is the reason behind the increased chemosis rates in the series of lower eyelid blepharoplasty utilizing lateral canthal support and re-draping of the orbicularis retaining ligament.[9,20,21]

This is particularly important when surgical procedures on the lower eyelid are combined with revolumization procedures in the malar region or nasojugal fold. Our studies would suggest that the key lymphatic drainage pathways for the lower eyelid are in close proximity to the nasojugal fold medially and the ORL, prezygomatic space, and malar fat pad laterally. Adjuvant filling of these areas should therefore only be undertaken with extreme care should concomitant lower eyelid surgery also be proposed.

Table 2.1 Rates of chemosis with different techniques of lower eyelid blepharoplasty

Author (Year)	Surgical technique	No. of patients	Chemosis rates
Seitz et al (2012)[18]	Transconjunctival deep midface lift	124	0.8%
Honrado et al (2004)[8]	Skin–muscle flap suspension suture	3988	1%
Prischmann et al (2013)[9]	Transconjunctival	39	5.1%
Undavia et al (2015)[19]	Transconjunctival	66	7.6%
Weinfeld et al (2008)[20]	Skin–muscle flap Release ORL Lateral canthopexy/plasty	312	11.5%
Codner et al (2008)[21]	Skin–muscle flap Release ORL Lateral canthopexy/plasty	264	12.1%
Prischmann et al (2013)[9]	Skin–muscle flap Lateral canthopexy	694	34.5%

Abbreviation: ORL, orbital retaining ligament.

References

1. Sappey MPC. Anatomie, physiologie, pathologie des vaisseaux lymphatiques consideres chez l'homme et les vertebres. Anatomie, Physiologie, Pathologie des Vaisseaux Lymphatiques Consideres Chez l'Homme et les Vertebres; 1874
2. Kinmonth JB. Lymphangiography in man; a method of outlining lymphatic trunks at operation. Clin Sci 1952;11(1):13–20
3. Suami H, Taylor GI, Pan WR. A new radiographic cadaver injection technique for investigating the lymphatic system. Plast Reconstr Surg 2005;115(7):2007–2013
4. Thompson JF, Uren RF, Shaw HM, et al. Location of sentinel lymph nodes in patients with cutaneous melanoma: new insights into lymphatic anatomy. J Am Coll Surg 1999;189(2):195–204
5. Tourani SS, Taylor GI, Ashton MW. Understanding the three-dimensional anatomy of the superficial lymphatics of the limbs. Plast Reconstr Surg 2014;134(5):1065–1074
6. Pan WR, Suami H, Taylor GI. Lymphatic drainage of the superficial tissues of the head and neck: anatomical study and clinical implications. Plast Reconstr Surg 2008;121(5):1614–1624, discussion 1625–1626
7. Pan WR, Le Roux CM, Briggs CA. Variations in the lymphatic drainage pattern of the head and neck: further anatomic studies and clinical implications. Plast Reconstr Surg 2011;127(2):611–620
8. Honrado CP, Pastorek NJ. Long-term results of lower-lid suspension blepharoplasty: a 30-year experience. Arch Facial Plast Surg 2004;6(3):150–154
9. Prischmann J, Sufyan A, Ting JY, Ruffin C, Perkins SW. Dry eye symptoms and chemosis following blepharoplasty: a 10-year retrospective review of 892 cases in a single-surgeon series. JAMA Facial Plast Surg 2013;15(1):39–46
10. Mendelson B, Wong C. Anatomy of the Ageing Face. In: Warren RJ NP, ed. Plastic Surgery. 2. 3rd ed. Elsevier; 2012
11. Rohrich RJ, Pessa JE. The fat compartments of the face: anatomy and clinical implications for cosmetic surgery. Plast Reconstr Surg 2007;119(7):2219–2227, discussion 2228–2231
12. Shoukath S, Taylor GI, Mendelson BC, Corlett RJ, Tourani SS, Shayan R, Ashton MW. The lymphatic anatomy of the lower eyelid and conjunctiva and correlation with postoperative chemosis and edema. Plast Reconstr Surg 2017;139(3):628e–637e
13. Hamra ST. Composite rhytidectomy. Plast Reconstr Surg 1992;90(1):1–13
14. Meade RA, Teotia SS, Griffeth LK, Barton FE. Facelift and patterns of lymphatic drainage. Aesthet Surg J 2012;32(1):39–45
15. Bähr W, Bagambisa FB, Schlegel G, Schilli W. Comparison of transcutaneous incisions used for exposure of the infraorbital rim and orbital floor: a retrospective study. Plast Reconstr Surg 1992;90(4):585–591
16. Mendelson BC, Muzaffar AR, Adams WP Jr. Surgical anatomy of the midcheek and malar mounds. Plast Reconstr Surg 2002;110(3):885–896, discussion 897–911
17. Slavin SA, Upton J, Kaplan WD, Van den Abbeele AD. An investigation of lymphatic function following free-tissue transfer. Plast Reconstr Surg 1997;99(3):730–741, discussion 742–743
18. Seitz IA, Llorente O, Few JW. The transconjunctival deep-plane midface lift: a 9-year experience working under the muscle. Aesthet Surg J 2012;32(6):692–699
19. Undavia S, Briceno CA, Massry GG. Quantified incision placement for postseptal approach transconjunctival blepharoplasty. Ophthal Plast Reconstr Surg 2016;32(3):191–194
20. Weinfeld AB, Burke R, Codner MA. The comprehensive management of chemosis following cosmetic lower blepharoplasty. Plast Reconstr Surg 2008;122(2):579–586
21. Codner MA, Wolfli JN, Anzarut A. Primary transcutaneous lower blepharoplasty with routine lateral canthal support: a comprehensive 10-year review. Plast Reconstr Surg 2008;121(1):241–250

Chapter 3

The Perioral Area, the Chin, and the Jowl

3 The Perioral Area, the Chin, and the Jowl

Jerome Paul Lamb, Christopher Chase Surek, and James D. Vargo

The Aging Characteristics of the Lip and Perioral Region: Contemporary Concepts

As far as we can tell, the perioral region is the one anatomical subunit of the face where muscle transformation plays a significant role in aging characteristics and appearance. Studies such as Iblher et al. and Penna et al. correlating radiographic change of soft and hard tissues to photometric changes offer the greatest insight into our understanding of the aging lip. Specifically, lengthening of the prolabium and loss of visible vermillion height are pathognomonic for an aging lip. Magnetic resonance imaging (MRI) scans demonstrate a decrease in anterior-posterior (A-P) dimension and increase in length without overall volume loss. Histomorphometric analysis demonstrates statistically significant thinning of the cutis, thickening of the subcutis, and a degeneration of elastic and collagen fibers.

The orbicularis oris muscle, which is composed of a pars marginalis and a pars peripheralis, becomes thinner with age (**Fig. 3.1**). As a result of pars marginalis descent, the muscle flattens and loses the forward curve (hockey stick) shape that is present in the youthful lip. This forward curve in the youthful lip is responsible for defining the vermillion border and consequently as the muscle changes with age the vermillion becomes less defined. In addition to soft-tissue changes, bony resorption of the anterior nasal spine and alveolus results in loss of anterior upper lip support, resulting in alterations to SNA measurements. Contrary to the upper lip, aging changes occurring in the lower lip are less quantified at present.

Deep Anatomy of the Chin and Jowl: The Mandibular Osseocutaneous Ligament and the Platysma Mandibular Ligament

There are two key retaining ligaments in the jowl. The inferior and superior superficial jowl compartments are separated from the more caudal submandibular fat compartment by a defined osseomuscular septum titled the platysma mandibular ligament (PML) or mandibular septum (**Fig. 3.2**). The PML is located approximately 5 cm distal to the gonial angle just above the mandibular border. It is postulated that this septum acts as "hammock" and physiologic laxity in its structural integrity leads to descent of jowl fat. The encasement of the PML with vascular channels likens it to a septum rather than a ligament. In addition, the PML is a point of muscular stability for the platysma as it glides over the mandible during coordinated movement, a function analogous to the orbital retaining ligament in the midface.

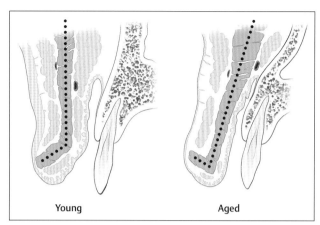

Fig. 3.1 Illustration representing the cross-sectional anatomy in the youthful and aged upper lip. Note the altered shape of the orbicularis oris muscle with age. The muscle flattens and loses the forward curve (hockey stick) shape that it possesses in the youthful lip. Adapted from Iblher N, Kloepper J, Penna V, Bartholomae JP, Stark GB. Changes in the aging upper lip—a photomorphometric and MRI-based study (on a quest to find the right rejuvenation approach). J Plast Reconstr Aesthet Surg 2008;61(10):1170–1176, Iblher N, Stark GB, Penna V. The aging perioral region—do we really know what is happening? J Nutr Health Aging 2012;16(6):581–585, and Penna V, Stark GB, Eisenhardt SU, Bannasch H, Iblher N. The aging lip: a comparative histological analysis of age-related changes in the upper lip complex. Plast Reconstr Surg 2009;124(2):624–628

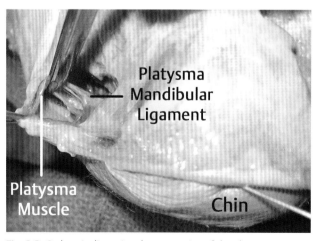

Fig. 3.2 Cadaveric dissection demonstration of the platysma mandibular ligaments.

Cephalic to the PML lies the mandibular osseocutaneous ligament (MOCL; **Fig. 3.3**). MOCL sits approximately 5.6 cm from the gonial angle and 1 cm above the mandibular border. The ligament spans 3.6 mm in width and its distal fibers interdigitate with the depressor anguli oris (DAO), forming inferior quadrant of the marionette lines. The MOCL can be palpated clinically as the tethering point between the anterior jowl and marionette line. This gives credence to the well-documented benefit of releasing this ligament for skin mobilization in rhytidectomy. In reference to the location of the mandibular ligament, recent literature confirms the position of the ligament to be at the anterior margin of the jowl, near the parasymphyseal region. Of note, the PML and MOCL are not to be confused with the masseteric cutaneous ligaments, which are nonosseous ligaments attaching muscle to overlying skin.

As the marginal mandibular nerve exits the parotid masseteric fascia, it travels sub-SMAS (subsuperficial muscular aponeurotic system) crossing the facial vessels 2.3 cm distal to the gonial angle. As the nerve crosses the vessels, it is 3 mm anterior to the vessel. The nerve does not transition superficially until it reaches the DAO. On average, the nerve will end as two branches with the dominant terminal branch ending 1 cm superior to the MOCL. Note that in accordance with traditional teaching, 81% of the time the nerve travels cranial to the mandibular border.

Injection Pearl

Injections caudal to the labiomental crease are SAFE.

Injection Pearl

Preperiosteal injections on the mandibular border are safe from a medial approach.

Fig. 3.4 shows the gross anatomy of the key retaining ligaments of the perioral region.

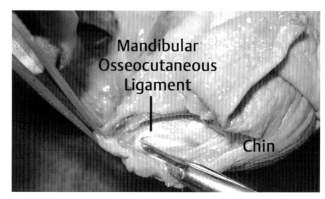

Fig. 3.3 Cadaveric dissection demonstration of the mandibular osseocutaneous ligament.

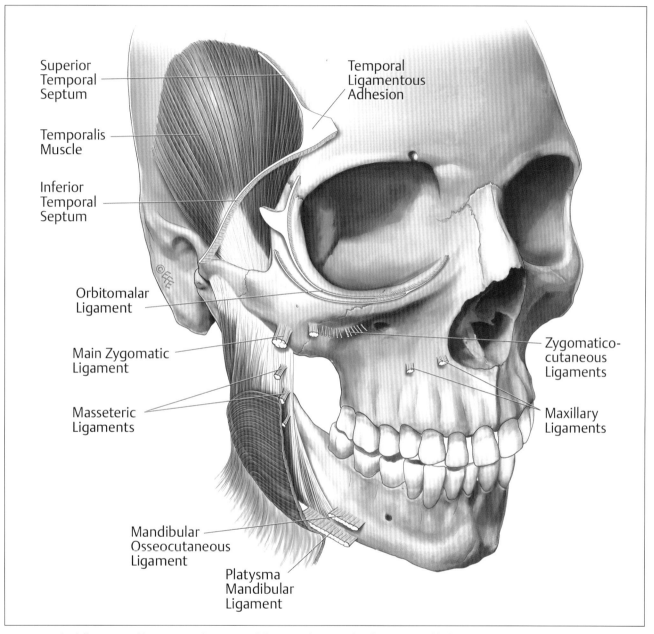

Superior Temporal Septum

Temporalis Muscle

Inferior Temporal Septum

Orbitomalar Ligament

Main Zygomatic Ligament

Masseteric Ligaments

Mandibular Osseocutaneous Ligament

Platysma Mandibular Ligament

Temporal Ligamentous Adhesion

Zygomatico-cutaneous Ligaments

Maxillary Ligaments

Fig. 3.4 Medical illustration of key retaining ligaments of the perioral region: the platysma mandibular ligament and the mandibular osseocutaneous ligament.

The Muscular and Compartment Anatomy of the Perioral Region

Muscular Anatomy

The three-dimensional (3D) muscular anatomy of the perioral region has been studied by Olzewski et al., but suffers from an $n = 1$ sample size. In fairness, the study is a report of methodology and not meant to represent a study of anatomic variability. However, this 3D MRI isotopic study in vivo demonstrates that the perioral musculature has a unique architecture.

The orbicularis oris muscle is more circular at its lateral extent, than elliptical. The deep fibers of the orbicularis oris are a result of interlacing buccinator muscle fibers, whereas the superficial fibers of the orbicularis oris arise from a coalescence with the lip elevators and lip depressors. The levator anguli oris (LAO) inserts behind the buccinators. The levator labii superioris (LLS) lies immediately alongside the LAO. The zygomaticus major muscle abuts the lateral edge of a vertical component of the orbicularis oris muscle. Of note, a lamina propria exists within the lip sphincter located between the orbicularis muscle and mucosa.

The lower perioral region contains three key muscles. The depressor labii inferioris (DLI), DAO, and mentalis muscle (**Fig. 3.5**). The DLI muscle originates on the mandible between the symphysis and mental forearm and inserts on the orbicularis muscle and skin. The DAO originates on the mandibular tubercle where it is fused with the platysma and inserts onto the modiolus and the angle of the mouth. Literature regarding mentalis muscle is sparse. The mentalis muscle originates on the upper symphysis and mental fat compartments, the fibers traverse cephalic fanning outward and interdigitating with orbicularis oris and skin of the lower lip. The mentalis muscle has a **V**-shaped configuration. Added to the DLI, it forms an "**M**"-shaped configuration in the lower lip. Mentalis strain is largely the result of poor bony support within individuals with Angle's Class II occlusion or in individuals with atrophy of the mental fat

Deep Lateral Chin Compartment

In the lower lip and prejowl lies the deep lateral chin compartment (**Fig. 3.6**). This compartment is a key augmentation target for volumization of the prejowl sulcus. This fat pad lies deep to the DAO to facilitate muscle gliding with movement. This sub-DAO fat has a thin gliding membrane along its anterior surface and protects the mental nerve that has a superomedial course and often accompanies the inferior labial artery. The diameter of the inferior labial artery makes small needle injection in the sub-DAO region a moderately risky proposition. Accessing this fat compartment via a cannula placed in the small triangle bounded by the lateral border of the DLI, the medial border of the DAO, and the caudal border of the orbicularis oris with an inferolateral angulation can be an effective volumization technique (**Fig. 3.7**). Alternatively, the caudal half of this compartment may be accessed via a paramedian chin pad approach, passing caudal to the mental nerve foramen over periosteum of the mandible, traversing in a medial to lateral direction.

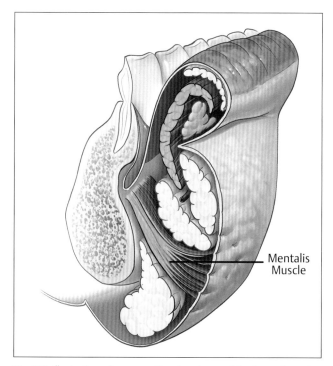

Fig. 3.5 Illustration of cross-sectional anatomy of the lower lip and chin, specifically the origin and insertion of the mentalis muscle. (Adapted from a medical illustration by James Vargo, MD.)

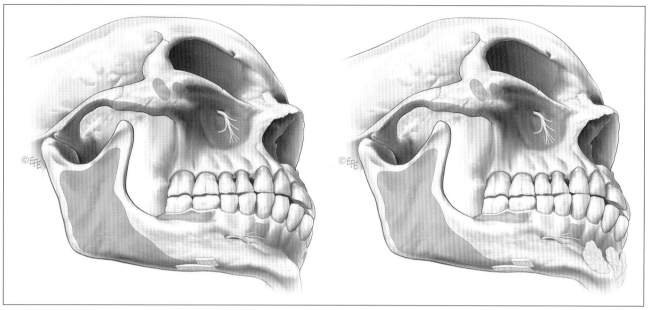

Fig. 3.6 Blue shading demonstrates origins and insertions of key perioral musculature. The mental fat pads are demonstrated.

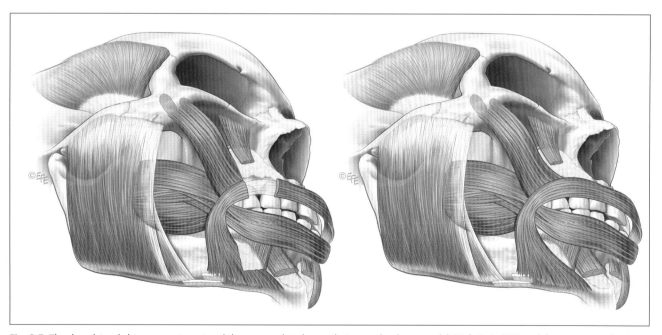

Fig. 3.7 The deep lateral chin compartment and the encapsulated space between the depressor labii inferioris (DLI) and depressor anguli oris (DAO) are demonstrated. Note the origin and insertion of the mentalis muscle along with the "M" configuration formed by the mentalis, DLI, and DAO.

Retro-orbicularis Oris Fat

Within the upper lip, a fibrofatty compartment exists deep to the orbicularis oris muscle, which appears to lose turgor with age. This retro-orbicularis oris fat (ROOrF) compartment has been briefly referenced by other authors who have studied perioral anatomy (**Fig. 3.8**). The caudal extent of the compartment is roughly the midpoint of the upper central dentition. The cephalad extent stops short of the labial buccal recess. Injection studies of the space freely flow superolateral to the orbicularis oris upper margin and progress from deep to superficial with the skin of the alar base and nasolabial fold. Clinically, we find this compartment to be a useful augmentation target in patients with upper alveolar collapse from previous bicuspid extraction, as well as pyriform aperture retrusion. The consistency of the fat is different than that of its cephalic counterparts. In cadaveric dissection, the fat is unfused with the overlying muscle and soft tissues and displays a sharp transition from its bordering structures outside the perioral aperture.

Superficial Lip Compartments

According to Pessa et al, the upper lip contains a series of superficial fat compartments (**Fig. 3.9**). These compartments are separated by vascularized septa containing arteries smaller than the outside diameter of 30-gauge needles, with the exception of the arteries coursing near or just slightly lateral to the philtral columns: the superior upper lip compartment, lateral upper lip compartment, inferior lateral upper lip compartment, and the central upper lip compartment. The central upper lip compartment contains an inferior and a superior quadrant. Clinically, these subcutaneous compartments are thin and compartmental division corresponds with vascular septation similar to other regions of the face. These septations are manifested as vertical perioral rhytids.

According to Pessa et al, the lower lip contains a trio of superficial fat compartments: the central lower lip fat compartment, lateral lip compartment, and the inferior chin compartment. The medial boundary of the lateral lip compartment is the septum containing the inferior labial artery. The arteries cephalic to the inferior labial–buccal sulcus are of the very small size, making intra-arterial cannulation by injection in these areas unlikely, and therefore render these compartments as potential targets for volumization.

Perioral Potential Spaces

Within the lower lip, a potential space exists over the ill-defined white roll. Arterial vasculature immediately deep to this space is intimate with the SMAS of the lower lip orbicularis oris. Cannula passage from commissure directed medially can easily traverse the entire lower lip. Cannula passage from a paramedian port, directed laterally, in this space finds a hard membranous barrier at the commissure and extending caudally a short distance.

Potential spaces also exist within the subvermillion of both the upper and lower lips. The upper lip has a potential space that is frequently medially partitioned posterior to the wet dry junction and a second space that is rarely partitioned anterior to the wet dry junction. The lower lip has a subvermillion space that is present both anterior and posterior to the wet–dry junction. The anterior space extends across the entire width of the lip and the posterior space ends at a midline partition.

The gross anatomy of the ROOrF is shown in **Fig. 3.10**, and **Fig. 3.11** depicts the superficial fat compartments of the perioral region.

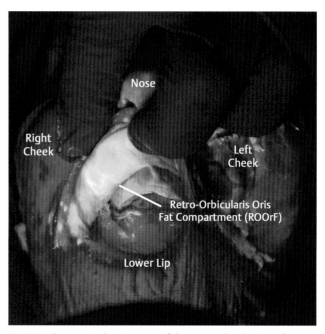

Fig. 3.8 Fluorescein dye injection of the retro-orbicularis oris fat (ROOrF) under black light illumination. Please note the rectangular shape of this structure.

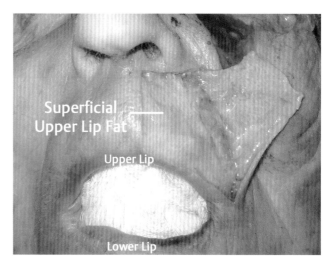

Fig. 3.9 Cadaveric dissection of the superficial upper lip fat compartment. Note the transition of loosely organized fat into a more fibrofatty composition. This line of fusion becomes more prominent with age.

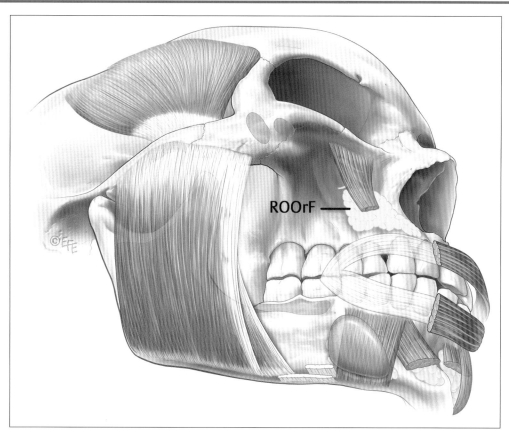

Fig. 3.10 Demonstration of the retro-orbicularis oris fat compartment.

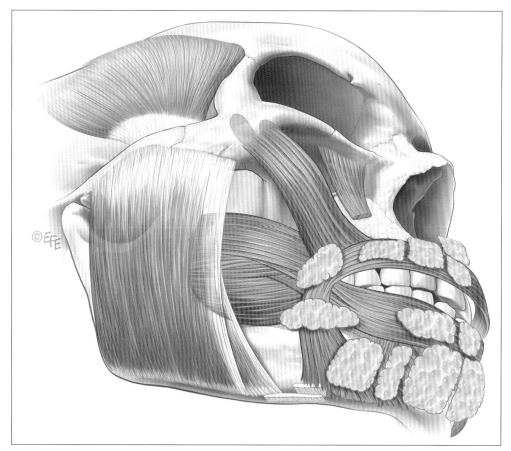

Fig. 3.11 Demonstration of the superficial upper and lower lip fat compartments.

Vascular Anatomy of the Lower Perioral Region

Understanding the architecture and blood supply in the lip and nasolabial region is critical to avoid unwanted complications. By standard definition, the facial artery ascends above the mandible deep to the platysma muscle branching into an inferior labial artery, superior labial artery (SLA), and continuing past the corner of the mouth toward the nose as the angular artery.

However, the variation in the patterns and locations of the facial artery branches has proven to be the rule and not the exception. Beginning in the neck, the facial artery will either bifurcate or give off the submental artery branch. Computed tomography angiography (CTA) studies have correlated the dominance of the facial artery at this bifurcation with the presence or absence of an angular system on the ipsilateral side. At this level, the average diameter of the vessel is approximately 2.3 mm. The vessel will travel deep to the DAO and zygomaticus major. This creates a safe harbor for any superficial injections done from commissure to nasolabial crease (**Fig. 3.12**).

Injection Pearl

Superficial injections in the region between the oral commissure and nasolabial crease are safe.

Studies have shown that often the inferior labial artery is ipsilaterally present and/or dominant, more commonly on the right than on the left side. The inferior labial artery passes deep to the platysma and generally forms a common trunk with the labiomental artery (**Fig. 3.13**). The labiomental artery has previously been referred to as the sublabial artery. The origin of the inferior labial artery lies within an area 2.4 cm from the labial commissure and 2.4 cm superior to the inferior edge of the mandible. The average vessel diameter at the ILA origin is 1.3 mm; the vessel traverses submucosal on the anterior wall of the oral cavity just above the mucosal attachment on the alveolar border. Some authors advocate the inferior border of the buccinator as an estimate of the level at which the ILA courses toward the midline. For topographic comparison, the ILA has predominately been shown to run as low as the labiomental crease. Unlike its cephalic counterpart, the ILA has been shown to run within the orbicularis muscle or between the orbicularis and lip depressors.

Often a sizable branch of the ILA will course with the mental nerve and the vessel will send small perpendicular perforators to the lower lip. As note of caution, a small percentage of ILA vessels will share a common trunk with the SLA before bifurcating; when this occurs, the ILA will run along the vermil-

lion–cutaneous junction. The incidence of this anomaly is approximately 11%. This can be problematic for needle injections along the vermillion–cutaneous junction and when placing boluses in the oral commissure. To date, studies are inconsistent in the depth of the ILA; as a general rule, the vessel is 4.7 mm deep at its origin and will transcend to 2.3 mm in depth upon reaching the midline.

Fig. 3.14 illustrates the vascular and fat compartment anatomy of the perioral region.

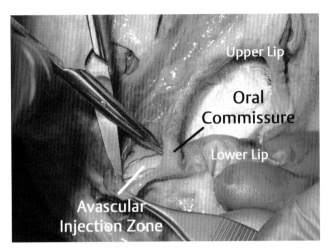

Fig. 3.12 Cadaveric dissection demonstration of safe injection zone in the oral commissure.

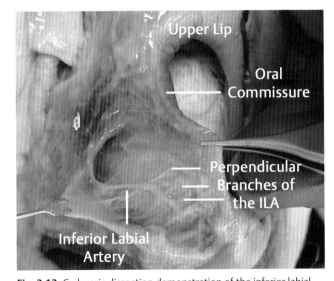

Fig. 3.13 Cadaveric dissection demonstration of the inferior labial artery.

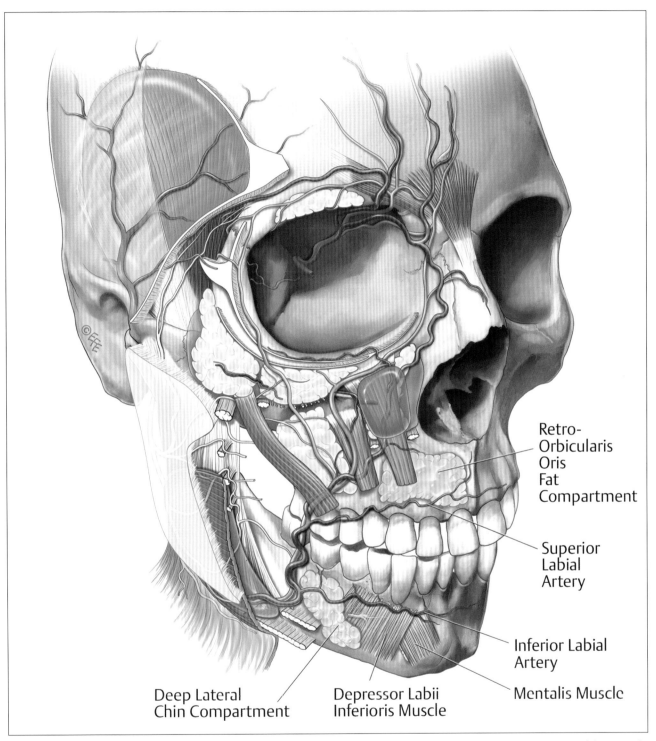

Fig. 3.14 Medical illustration of sub-SMAS (subsuperficial muscular aponeurotic system) vascular and fat compartment anatomy of the perioral region.

Vascular Anatomy of the Upper Lip and the Superficial Fat Compartments

The SMAS of the lip has been previously described by Pensler et al. The facial nerve innervation of the orbicularis oris muscle of the upper lip enters superior laterally on the underside of the muscle and has numerous small branches. Recent studies have delineated the topographic location of the SLA. Lee et al categorize the branching pattern of the SLA into four types. According to this cadaver study, approximately 22% of superior labial arteries will provide the ipsilateral alar branch. Presumably in the remaining 78% of specimens, the angular or infraorbital vessels supply the alar branch. In addition, this study found that the superior labial vessel is absent on one side in 7% of specimens.

Computed tomography studies have reported an incidence of up to 43% of subjects where the SLA was not present bilaterally. The takeoff of the SLA has been isolated to a 1.5 cm² area from the oral commissure with a depth location of approximately 3.5 mm (**Figs. 3.15**, **3.16**). Clinically, the injector can place his/her thumbnail at the oral commissure to estimate vessel location. The SLA pierces the orbicularis oris muscle and then travels cephalically to the vermillion cutaneous border until it reaches a relative midpoint between the oral commissure and the ipsilateral cupid bow peak, at which time it will descend below the white roll and continue to the sagittal midline. This transition zone is important knowledge for the injector when performing upper lip injections. At the level of the Cupid's bow peak, the SLA is approximately 1 mm inferior to the cutaneous vermillion border. During its entire course, the SLA maintains a depth of at least 3 mm. Upon approaching the midline, 85% of SLA systems have a septal branch, the majority of septal branches will ascend to the nose in a suborbicularis plane; however, up to 25% of branches will travel superficial to the muscle. This is a consideration to be noted when performing philtral injections, as embolization of these vessels can lead to nasal tissue loss.

Injection Pearl

"2-4-5" Rule for Lip Injection. The SLA runs 2 mm anterior to the intraoral mucosa, at least 4 mm deep to the skin, and is 5 mm in depth centrally at the lower lip margin.

Superficial Lip Compartments

As previously mentioned, Pessa et al describe a series of superficial upper lip fat compartments (**Fig. 3.17**): the superior upper lip compartment, lateral upper lip compartment, inferior lateral upper lip compartment, and the central upper lip compartment. The central upper lip compartment contains an inferior and a superior quadrant. Clinically, these subcutaneous compartments are thin and compartmental division corresponds with vascular septation similar to other regions of the face. These septations are manifested as vertical perioral rhytids. The lower lip contains a trio of superficial fat compartments: the central lower lip fat compartment, lateral lip compartment, and the inferior chin compartment. The medial boundary of the lateral lip compartment is the septum containing the inferior labial artery. The arteries cephalic to the inferior labial–buccal

sulcus are of the very small size, making intra-arterial cannulation by injection in these areas unlikely, and therefore render these compartments as potential targets for volumization.

Fig. 3.18 shows the superficial fat compartments of the perioral region.

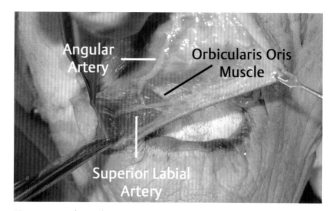

Fig. 3.15 Cadaver dissection demonstration of the superior labial artery.

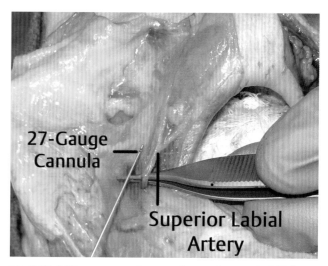

Fig. 3.16 A 27-gauge cannula comparison to the superior labial artery in a cadaveric specimen.

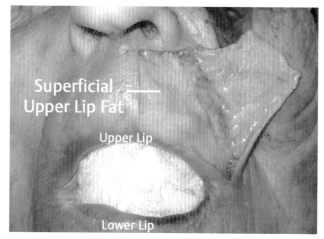

Fig. 3.17 Cadaveric dissection of the superficial upper lip fat compartment. Note the transition of loosely organized fat into a more fibrofatty composition. This line of fusion becomes more prominent with age.

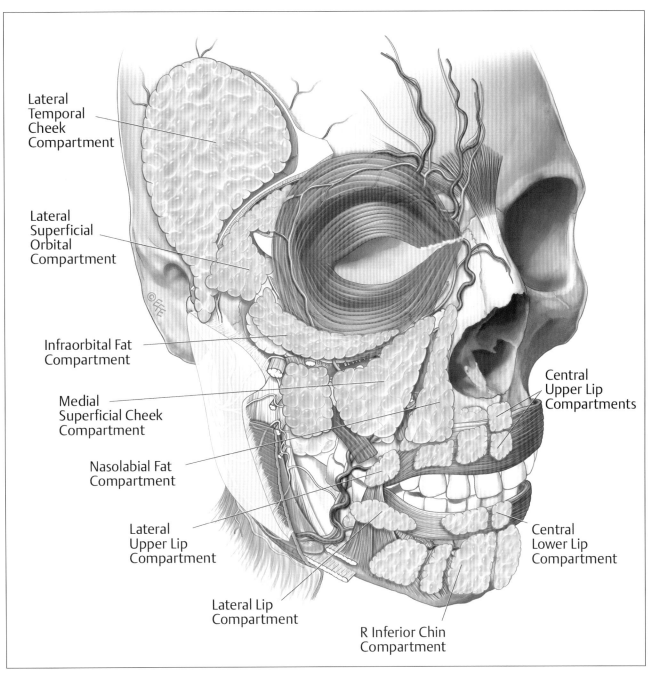

Lateral Temporal Cheek Compartment

Lateral Superficial Orbital Compartment

Infraorbital Fat Compartment

Medial Superficial Cheek Compartment

Nasolabial Fat Compartment

Lateral Upper Lip Compartment

Lateral Lip Compartment

Central Upper Lip Compartments

Central Lower Lip Compartment

R Inferior Chin Compartment

Fig. 3.18 Medical illustration of superficial fat compartments in the perioral region. These compartments are thin and compartmental division corresponds with vascular septation similar to other regions of the face. These septations are manifested as vertical perioral rhytids.

Nasolabial Anatomy

Moving cephalically into the nasolabial fold, studies indicate an intimate relationship of the facial artery to the nasolabial fold approaching 93%. Given the tortuous nature of the artery, it is difficult to provide concrete topographic mapping for the purpose of injections. Yang et al in a large cadaveric study provided data on location of depth of the artery relative to the fold. The artery more commonly travels medial to the fold, starting 1.7 mm medial from the fold in the lower portion and crossing beneath the fold at a depth of 5 mm at the superior third of the fold, eventually reaching a point 3.2 cm lateral to the nasal ala.

Cadaveric dissection has revealed insertion of the LLSAN, LLS, and zygomaticus minor into the nasolabial fold, and it is within these muscle fibers that the artery traverses medial to lateral across the fold. This knowledge of muscular insertion has led some authors to advocate for botulinum toxin injections into the nasolabial fold as alternative means for fold effacement (**Fig. 3.19**). Release of the dermal attachments of the mimetic muscles in the nasolabial fold is a well-established tenant in rhytidectomy. The knowledge of mimetic muscle relationship to the nasolabial fold supports the notion that volumizing the deep medial cheek fat and deep pyriform space can create a fulcrum lift of the lip elevators resulting in a softening of the nasolabial fold restoring youthful appearance to the face (**Videos 3.1, 3.2**).

Injection Pearl

When injecting the nasolabial fold, we recommend needle placement in the reticular dermis or immediate subcutis. Be cognizant of the depth of the angular artery (~5 mm) and the level at which it crosses the nasolabial fold (junction of the proximal third). To confirm depth, the injector should see the white color of blanching skin, but NOT the gray color of the needle. If the injector sees the gray of the needle, the needle location is too superficial and should be readjusted. The authors recommend gentle needle subcision of the fold followed by retrograde injection of medium-sized hyaluronic acid (HA) filler.

As discussed earlier in this chapter, the ROOrF lies immediately deep to the orbicularis oris muscle overlying the canine fossa (**Fig. 3.20**). This compartment is an excellent target for upper lip volume replenishment, particularly in patients with upper alveolar collapse from prior bicuspid extractions incidental to orthodontic manipulation (see section "Authors' Preferred Technique for Perioral Rejuvenation")

Fig. 3.21 shows the gross anatomy of the structures that lie beneath the nasolabial fold and the perioral skin.

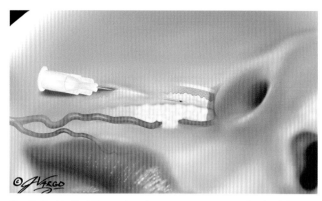

Fig. 3.19 Medical illustration demonstrating proper depth of the needle insertion for nasolabial fold filler injection. (Adapted from a medical illustration by James Vargo, MD.)

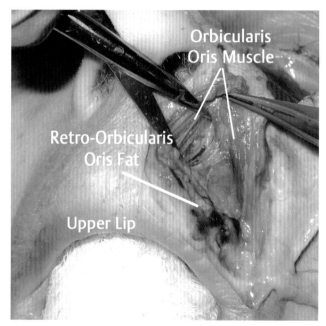

Fig. 3.20 Cadaveric dissection demonstration of the retro-orbicularis oris fat (ROOrF) compartment. The compartment was percutaneously injected with hyaluronic acid homogenized with green dye prior to dissection.

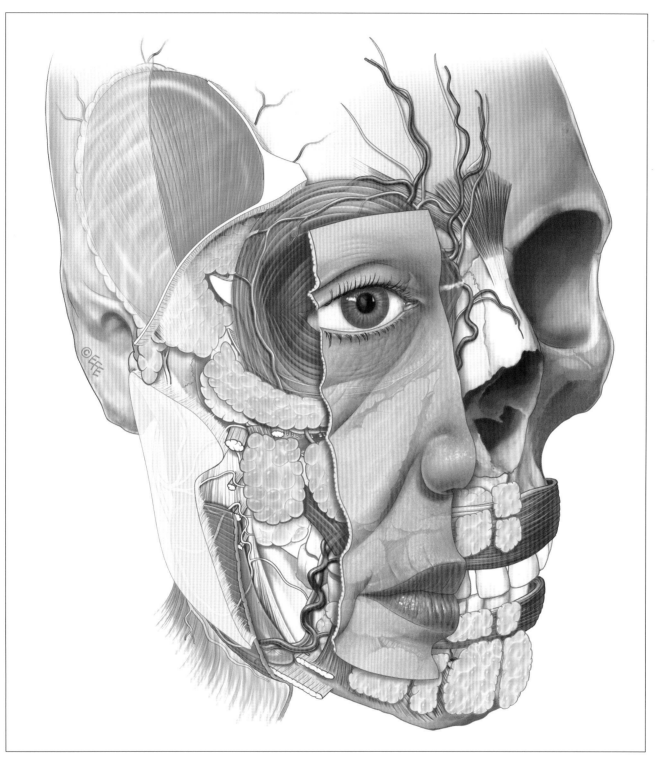

Fig. 3.21 Medical illustration of demonstrating the nasolabial fold and perioral skin with demonstration of underlying anatomic structures.

The Authors' Preferred Techniques for Perioral Rejuvenation

Columella–Lip Interface

Retro-Orbicularis Oris Fat

In perioral rejuvenation, the determination is first made regarding dental occlusion. In individuals who have undergone orthodontic extractions of upper first bicuspids, generally a broad level of upper lip collapse will be present. The ROOrF represents a volumizable compartment for both autologous fat grafting and/or off-the-shelf fillers. This fat compartment extends to the junction of the middle third of the vertical height of the upper lip and extends medially to the entrance of the deep-pyriform space. This fat compartment is devoid of arteries large enough to be cannulated readily. The authors' preferred technique is to approach this compartment with a port placed centrally in the philtrum at the junction of the upper third of the philtrum (see illustration). The injector begins with a small "wheel" bolus within the port using a small amount of Xylocaine with epinephrine to minimize bruising (**Video 3.3**). A cannula is passed through the port in an anterior to posterior direction; the cannula is then angulated laterally and easily runs on the anterior side of the upper lip mucosa, deep to the orbicularis oris muscle. The cannula encounters very little restriction in this potential space. When using off-the-shelf HA fillers, the fillers are blended with a 2:1 ratio of filler to Xylocaine. Approximately 0.4 mL of the blended product is injected per side. Injection of the ROOrF through this central cannula approach with hyaluronic filler will permeate the more areolar fat that is present in the upper outer triangle of the upper lip bordering the alar cheek junction (**Fig. 3.22**; **Video 3.4**). When grafting autologous fat, the fat is placed in numerous passes, while the cannula is passed in a fan-shaped manner. In summary, volumization of these suborbicularis oris structures broadens the dental arch and often lifts the upper lip.

Vertical Perioral Rhytids

Vertical perioral rhytids within the lower third of the upper lip are generally not the purview of autologous fat grafting procedures. When present, the authors prefer primarily crosshatching in an intradermal level with particulate HA products (**Video 3.5**). Prior to injection, the product is transferred to a 1-mL Luer-Lock syringe, which will break the particle into a smaller size. A 32-gauge needle is used for the injection. Alternatively, HA fillers designed to avoid a Tyndell effect may be placed in the subcutaneous fat of the upper lip over the course of the orbicularis oris muscle.

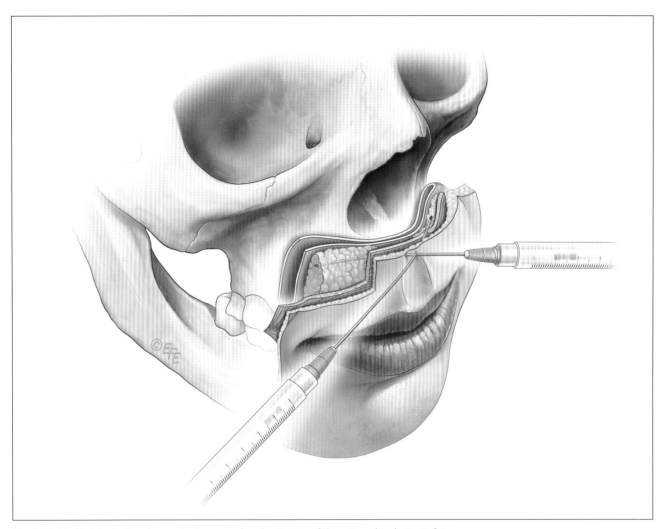

Fig. 3.22 Medical illustration demonstrating cannula volumization of the retro-orbicularis oris fat.

Upper Lip Enhancement

The Philtrum and the White Roll

The philtrum is injected immediately subdermal through a white roll approach (**Fig. 3.23**; **Video 3.6**). The philtrum is gently pinched between the injector's nondominant thumb and index finger, which lifts the tissue away from potential ascending branches of the SLA. The white roll is enhanced from commissure to commissure including the philtral component with HA filler using a 30-gauge needle while pressing the white roll between thumb and index finger and injecting upon withdrawal. A very sharp and unexaggerated white roll can be achieved in this fashion. Enhancement of the white roll should precede any vermillion enhancements.

The Oral Commissure

Although it has not been studied photomicrographically, the lower lip adjacent to the commissure is conjectured to be composed of fibrofatty tissue that, with age, becomes atrophic or misshapen. Depressed lateral commissures are addressed by an injection of HA filler superficially into the caudal aspect of the orbicularis oris muscle approximately 5 mm lateral to the commissure creating a downward curvature at this 5-mm point. The injection is placed superficial, intramuscular, and falls both anterior and caudal to the course of the SLA. By proxy, this maneuver results in the illusion of an upturned commissure (**Video 3.7**).

The Red Vermillion

One method for enhancement of the dry vermilion is accomplished through a "no touch" vertical needle injection in the white roll where HA filler is placed in an anteroposterior direction immediately deep to the dry vermillion mucosa. Parallel injections at approximately 1.5- to 2-mm increments in the central three-quarters of the upper lip vermillion are performed from commissure to commissure. This method will result in maximal vermilion convexity and improved anteroposterior projection of the red lip. The needle must not be angulated in a posterosuperior direction as this increases the likelihood of an intra-arterial injection into the SLA.

An alternative method to augment the red vermilion is via cannula (**Videos 3.8**). Two potential spaces exist within the upper lip subvermillion. One lies anterior to the wet–dry junction and the second lies posterior. The anterior space extends the entire width of the upper lip in most individuals, whereas the posterior space is partitioned at the midline in most individuals. A port is made just lateral to the commissure. The injector places a small bolus of Xylocaine with epinephrine for minimization of bleeding and bruising. The cannula may then be passed in both spaces to provide increased projection of the dry vermillion and increased height of the wet vermillion, respectively. This can assist in restoring upper lip projection relative to the lower lip in a profile view, along with decreasing excessive gingival show.

The anatomical shape of the orbicularis oris has a vertical component of its fibers at the commissure. This transition from transverse to vertical leaves an area of poor soft-tissue support, resulting in oral incompetence, in both the upper and the lower lips. The superior and inferior labial arteries are not in close proximity to this area deficiency. Oral competence is best achieved from a medial to lateral injection at and just slightly posterior to the white roll of the upper and lower lip commissure (**Video 3.9**).

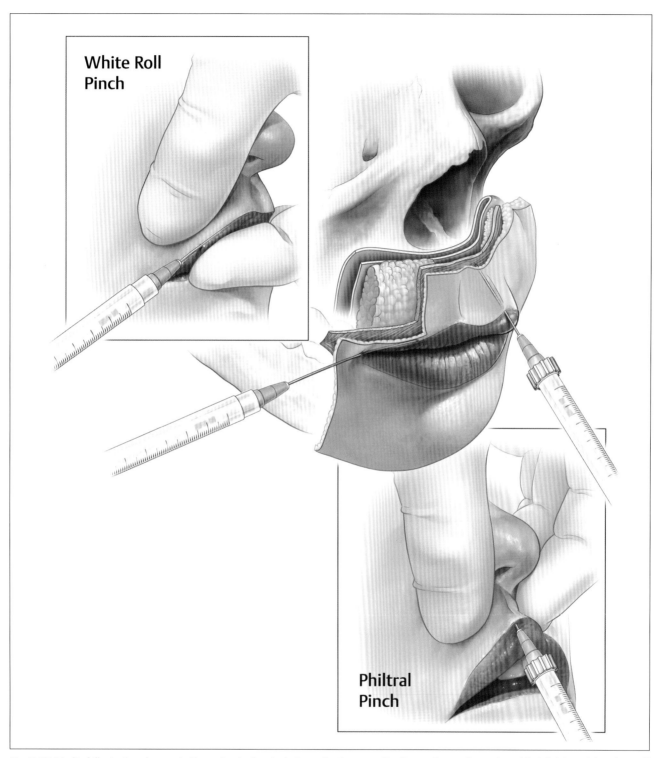

White Roll Pinch

Philtral Pinch

Fig. 3.23 Medical illustration demonstrating volumization techniques for the upper lip. Our preference is starting with definition of the white roll and philtrum and then progressing to vermillion enhancement. For philtral injection, 29- to 30-gauge 0.5-in needles are used.

Lower Lip Enhancement

Similar to the upper lip, two methods can be utilized to enhance the white roll: cannula or needle. Our preferred method is to use a cannula as we find the cannula stays nicely centered on the white roll (**Videos 3.10, 3.11**). Using an oral commissure insertion point, a retrograde cannula injection spanning the white vermillion can also be performed. Sequential needle injections can be performed with HA filler using a 30-gauge needle while pressing the white roll between thumb and index finger and injecting upon withdrawal.

Needle enhancement of the dry vermilion is accomplished through a "no touch" vertical needle injection in the white roll where HA filler is placed in an anteroposterior direction immediately deep to the dry vermillion mucosa (**Fig. 3.24**). Parallel injections at approximately 1.5- to 2-mm increments in the central three-quarters of the lower lip vermilion are performed from commissure to commissure. This method will result in maximal vermilion convexity and improved anteroposterior projection of the red lip. The needle must not be angulated in a posteroinferior direction as this increases the likelihood of an intra-arterial injection into the vertical branches of the inferior labial artery.

For lower lip vermillion enhancement with cannula, the injector can utilize the same cannula port that was used in the upper lip. The cannula can be angulated caudally into a space beneath the anterior vermilion of the lower lip. This space transverses the entire lower lip.

The lower lip contribution to the commissure is addressed by injecting the superficial lateral fat compartment of the lower lip, which in many individuals is a tightly bound compartment. Excessive injection within this space will result in a deformity, which looks unnatural. The marionette line exists where a thicker fat compartment laterally abuts more thin compartments medially. Crosshatching with immediate subdermal injections is effective on the marionette lines. The injector should make an assessment of concavities over the DAO muscle. Cannula injections with HA filler or autologous fat over the DAO should be done conservatively; however, as all vascularity runs deep to the DAO, superficial injections are safe to perform in this region.

Soft-tissue atrophy in the lower lip superficial fat compartments occurs and should be assessed. Superficial injections in the lower lip are safe and easy to perform with a cannula with either a midline chin port or a port at the lateral extent of the labiomental crease.

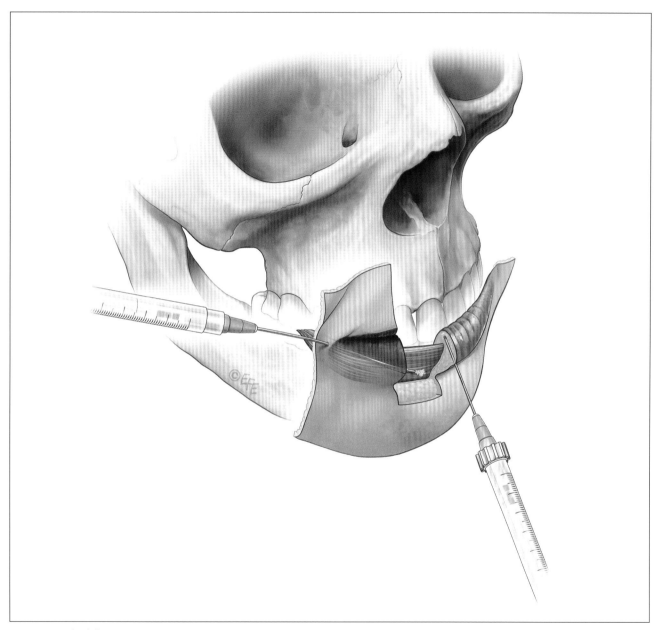

Fig. 3.24 Medical illustration demonstrating volumization techniques for the lower lip. Cannula volumization of the vermillion is depicted. Needle "no touch" approach with vertical injections deep to dry vermillion is depicted. For this technique, 29- to 30-gauge 0.5-in needles are preferred.

Lip–Chin Interface

Support for the lower lip and chin interface is achieved by restoring volume within the area of the labiomental crease (**Fig. 3.25**). The inferior labial artery runs in close proximity to the labial–buccal sulcus on the deep side of the lower lip. Injections performed with the cannula from a central port will find a natural plane. Volume is added over the cephalic insertion of the mentalis muscle along the posterior aspect of the orbicularis oris muscle and more laterally over the DLI. Injection should be superficial (i.e., subcutaneous) to add support and minimize intravascular complications.

When mentalis strain is present, volume should be placed in the mentalis fat pad, which is septated at the midline. A midline port at the point of maximal chin convexity can be utilized. Once subcutaneous, the injector can angulate the cannula slightly off the midline and will meet resistance just before the cannula enters the fat pad.

A cannula port along the inferior border of the mandible at the parasagittal midline facilitates cannula passage cephalically in a sub-DAO plane. In this location, the injector can volumize the deep lateral chin compartment and provide support deep and medial to the lower lip commissure. The cannula can be advanced laterally just above the mandibular border where it will meet very little resistance as it enters the deep lateral chin compartment; this potential space is formed by the investing capsule on the posterior surface of the DAO and volume can be placed in this space to provide support beneath the DAO. This injection target will assist in blending the jawline and camouflaging the prejowl (**Video 3.12**). Autologous fat and high G-prime off-the-shelf HA fillers can be used interchangeably with these approaches.

Additionally, the jowl can be camouflaged by superficial subcutaneous injections through a midline port without concern for intravascular injection. Immediate subcutaneous injections of the prejowl sulcus are equally safe with needle and cannula.

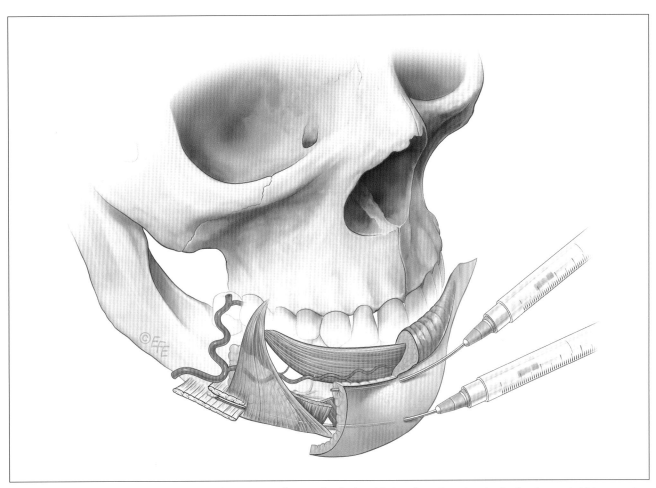

Fig. 3.25 Medical illustration demonstrating volumization techniques for the lip–chin interface. Cannula volumization the mental fat compartments and labiomental crease is demonstrated. Cannula volumization of the deep lateral chin compartment from a midline ports is demonstrated; the cannula is advanced on the backside of the depressor anguli oris.

Suggested Reading

Chin and Jowl Anatomy

Braz A, Humphrey S, Weinkle S, et al. Lower face: clinical anatomy and regional approaches with injectable fillers. Plast Reconstr Surg 2015; 136(5, Suppl):235S–257S

Cardoso ER, Amonoo-Kuofi HS, Hawary MB. Mentolabial sulcus: a histologic study. Int J Oral Maxillofac Surg 1995;24(2):145–147

de Castro CC. The anatomy of the platysma muscle. Plast Reconstr Surg 1980;66(5):680–683

Feldman J. Neck Lift. St. Louis, MO: Quality Medical Publishing, Inc.; 2006:107

Furnas DW. The retaining ligaments of the cheek. Plast Reconstr Surg 1989;83(1):11–16

Huettner F, Rueda S, Ozturk CN, et al. The relationship of the marginal mandibular nerve to the mandibular osseocutaneous ligament and lesser ligaments of the lower face. Aesthet Surg J 2015;35(2):111–120

Mendelson BC, Muzaffar AR, Adams WP Jr. Surgical anatomy of the midcheek and malar mounds. Plast Reconstr Surg 2002;110(3):885–896, discussion 897–911

Reece EM, Pessa JE, Rohrich RJ. The mandibular septum: anatomical observations of the jowls in aging-implications for facial rejuvenation. Plast Reconstr Surg 2008;121(4):1414–1420

Upper Lip

Crouzet C, Fournier H, Papon X, Hentati N, Cronier P, Mercier P. Anatomy of the arterial vascularization of the lips. Surg Radiol Anat 1998;20(4):273–278

Furukawa M, Mathes DW, Anzai Y. Evaluation of the facial artery on computed tomographic angiography using 64-slice multidetector computed tomography: implications for facial reconstruction in plastic surgery. Plast Reconstr Surg 2013;131(3):526–535

Iblher N, Kloepper J, Penna V, Bartholomae JP, Stark GB. Changes in the aging upper lip—a photomorphometric and MRI-based study (on a quest to find the right rejuvenation approach). J Plast Reconstr Aesthet Surg 2008;61(10):1170–1176

Iblher N, Stark GB, Penna V. The aging perioral region—do we really know what is happening? J Nutr Health Aging 2012;16(6):581–585

Lee SH, Gil YC, Choi YJ, Tansatit T, Kim HJ, Hu KS. Topographic anatomy of the superior labial artery for dermal filler injection. Plast Reconstr Surg 2015;135(2):445–450

Loukas M, Hullett J, Louis RG Jr, et al. A detailed observation of variations of the facial artery, with emphasis on the superior labial artery. Surg Radiol Anat 2006;28(3):316–324

Nakajima H, Imanishi N, Aiso S. Facial artery in the upper lip and nose: anatomy and a clinical application. Plast Reconstr Surg 2002;109(3):855–861, discussion 862–863

Olszewski R, Liu Y, Duprez T, Xu TM, Reychler H. Three-dimensional appearance of the lips muscles with three-dimensional isotropic MRI: in vivo study. Int J CARS 2009;4(4):349–352

Penna V, Stark GB, Eisenhardt SU, Bannasch H, Iblher N. The aging lip: a comparative histological analysis of age-related changes in the upper lip complex. Plast Reconstr Surg 2009;124(2):624–628

Pensler JM, Ward JW, Parry SW. The superficial musculoaponeurotic system in the upper lip: an anatomic study in cadavers. Plast Reconstr Surg 1985;75(4):488–494

Pinar YA, Bilge O, Govsa F. Anatomic study of the blood supply of perioral region. Clin Anat 2005;18(5):330–339

Surek CC, Guisantes E, Schnarr K, Jelks G, Beut J. "No touch" technique for lip enhancement. Plast Reconstr Surg 2016;138(4):603e–613e

Lower Lip

Edizer M, Mağden O, Tayfur V, Kiray A, Ergür I, Atabey A. Arterial anatomy of the lower lip: a cadaveric study. Plast Reconstr Surg 2003;111(7):2176–2181

Tansatit T, Apinuntrum P, Phetudom T. A typical pattern of the labial arteries with implication for lip augmentation with injectable fillers. Aesthetic Plast Surg 2014;38(6):1083–1089

Nasolabial Fold

Barton FE Jr, Gyimesi IM. Anatomy of the nasolabial fold. Plast Reconstr Surg 1997;100(5):1276–1280

Beer GM, Manestar M, Mihic-Probst D. The causes of the nasolabial crease: a histomorphological study. Clin Anat 2013;26(2):196–203

Pessa JE, Brown F. Independent effect of various facial mimetic muscles on the nasolabial fold. Aesthetic Plast Surg 1992;16(2):167–171

Rubin LR, Mishriki Y, Lee G. Anatomy of the nasolabial fold: the keystone of the smiling mechanism. Plast Reconstr Surg 1989;83(1):1–10

Yang HM, Lee JG, Hu KS, et al. New anatomical insights on the course and branching patterns of the facial artery: clinical implications of injectable treatments to the nasolabial fold and nasojugal groove. Plast Reconstr Surg 2014;133(5):1077–1082

Complication Management

Cohen JL. Understanding, avoiding, and managing dermal filler complications. Dermatol Surg 2008;34(Suppl 1):S92–S99

Daines SM, Williams EF. Complications associated with injectable soft-tissue fillers: a 5-year retrospective review. JAMA Facial Plast Surg 2013;15(3):226–231

DeLorenzi C. Complications of injectable fillers, part I. Aesthet Surg J 2013;33(4):561–575

DeLorenzi C. Complications of injectable fillers, part 2: vascular complications. Aesthet Surg J 2014;34(4):584–600

Eversole R, Tran K, Hansen D, Campbell J. Lip augmentation dermal filler reactions, histopathologic features. Head Neck Pathol 2013;7(3):241–249

Park TH, Seo SW, Kim JK, Chang CH. Clinical experience with hyaluronic acid-filler complications. J Plast Reconstr Aesthet Surg 2011;64(7):892–896

Sclafani AP, Fagien S. Treatment of injectable soft tissue filler complications. Dermatol Surg 2009;35(Suppl 2):1672–1680

Chapter 4

The Temple and the Brow

4 The Temple and the Brow

Jerome Paul Lamb and Christopher Chase Surek

The Temporal Fascia Layers, the Upper and Lower Temporal Compartments, and the Inferior Temporal Septum

Temple hallowing is a common problem in the aging face, and nomenclature can be confusing. Volume lost with aging in the temple may be the result of atrophy of the temple fat pad, superficial lateral orbital fat, and lateral temporal cheek fat. The coined term *temporal hollowing* reflects deficiency in the temporal adipose and/or muscle. In accordance with this aging phenomenon, the more prominent skeletal contours adjacent to the temple can further diminish the perceived projection of the temple. As a general rule, authors advocate undercorrection compared to overcorrection for temporal contour (**Video 4.1**).

As the scalp layers converge into the temple, the galea aponeurotica becomes the superficial temporal fascia (synonymous with the temporoparietal fascia [TPF]); in contrast, the periosteum becomes synonymous with the deep temporal fascia. The deep temporal fascia is composed of separately named lamina (superficial and deep) at the level of the zygomatic arch. These laminae will fuse 2 to 3 cm cephalic to the zygomatic arch into one layer at the temporal line of fusion. A reproducible method to understanding the temporal anatomy is to divide the temporal into upper and lower temporal compartments. This has been refined and well described by Bryan Mendelson and his colleagues.

The upper temporal compartment is bordered superiorly by the superior temporal septum. This septum is the upper limit of the temple region. It is at this point that the periosteum converts to deep temporal fascia. The septum traverses anteriorly to the triangular temporal ligamentous adhesion (TLA). The TLA is a "keystone" that represents the convergence of the superior and inferior temporal septa. No vital structures exist in the superior temporal compartment and it is within the bounds of this space that the surgical dissector can visualize the straddling of the temporal fat compartment by the two laminae of deep temporal fascia.

The lower temporal compartment cephalic border is the inferior temporal septum. The compartment floor is comprised of dense fibrofatty parotid temporal fascia; this fascia condenses as it travels caudally to the lower zygoma merging with the zygomaticocutaneous ligaments and forming the relative inferior border of the compartment.

The deep fat compartment of the upper periorbital region is the retro-orbicularis oculi fat (ROOF) compartment. The fat resides deep in the orbicularis oculi muscle and galea. Deflation of this fat results in deep upper eyelid sulci and descent of the tail of the eyebrow.

A thorough understanding of temple vascular anatomy is important to avoid undesirable complications. Three separate branches of the external carotid artery provide vascular supply within the temple region. The superficial temporal artery (STA) courses within the TPF. An anterior branch of the STA will run with the temporal rami of the facial nerve and often communicates with the supraorbital artery (**Fig. 4.1**). Intravascular injection of this artery can result is retrograde thrombosis of the ophthalmic system and subsequent central retinal artery occlusion and blindness; therefore, superficial needle injection in the region should be performed with caution. Within the deep temporal fascia lie the middle temporal and deep temporal arteries. Of note, the deep temporal artery arises from the internal maxillary artery. Inadvertent injection into this artery can result in retrograde vascular occlusion and significant complications. As a result, we only recommend needle injections in the inferior medial quadrant of the temporal fossa (see section "The Authors' Preferred Techniques for Temporal Volumization"). For the remainder of the temple, we recommend cannulas either in the upper temporal compartment, which is an avascular plane, or in the superficial temporal fat compartments.

Fig. 4.2 presents the gross anatomy of the neurovasculature and the upper temporal space.

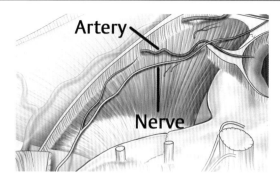

Fig. 4.1 Illustration of the intersection of the frontal branch of the facial nerve and anterior branch of the superficial temporal artery.

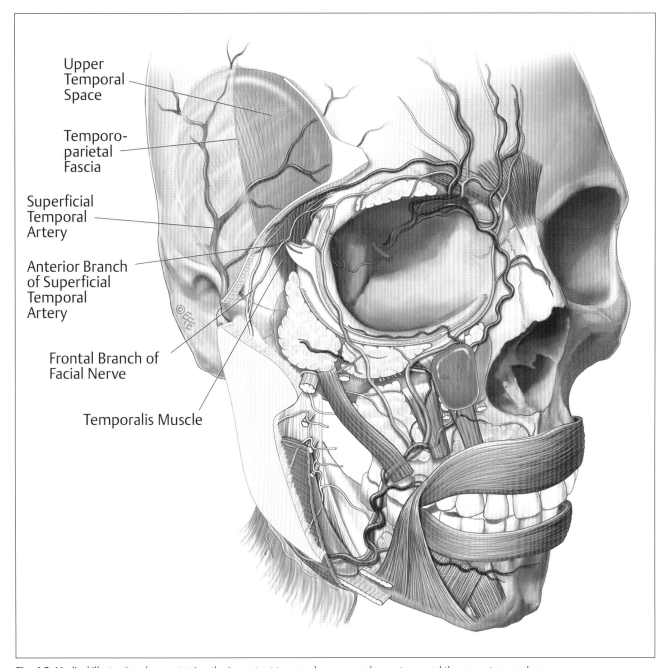

Fig. 4.2 Medical illustration demonstrating the important temporal neurovascular anatomy and the upper temporal space.

Upper
Temporal
Space

Temporo-
parietal
Fascia

Superficial
Temporal
Artery

Anterior Branch
of Superficial
Temporal
Artery

Frontal Branch of
Facial Nerve

Temporalis Muscle

The Superficial Temporal Artery, the Sentinel Vein, the Brow Partition, and the Superficial Temporal Components

The inferior temporal septum is a bilaminar ligamentous structure; the inferior lamina stabilizes the temporal rami branch of the facial nerve. This branch is synonymous with the frontal branch of the facial nerve. The frontal branch courses near the periosteum of the lateral zygomatic arch coursing anterior and inferior to the inframtemporal septum. The nerve becomes more superficial as it courses cephalic running in the TPF within the ceiling of the inferior temporal compartment. The frontal branch consistently crosses superficial to an anterior branch of the STA, where it is minimally invested by thin fascia immediately beneath the subcutaneous fat. These rami will continue their course into the forehead and ROOF. It is important to note that zygomaticotemporal branches and the sentinel vein course within the inferior temporal compartment. Cannula-based procedures readily glide along the superficial extension of the inframtemporal septum within the upper temporal space. Surgical augmentation with implants or other synthetic composites demonstrates that volumization can be performed in both submuscular and supramusclar planes in this compartment.

An additional anatomic structure of note is the temporal tunnel as defined by Bryan Mendelson. This is a deep space traversing between the lateral orbital thickening (superiorly), orbicularis retaining ligament (medially), and TPF (laterally). Blunt dissection through this space safely leads to the prezygomatic space.

There are two fat compartments in the temple region. The first is the superficial lateral temporal cheek fat compartment.

The cephalic border of this fat compartment is the temporal crest and the superior temporal septum; the compartment is a good target for temple volumization. Blunt cannulas will meet resistance at the caudal and cephalic boundaries of the compartment corresponding with the temporal septa as they insert into skin. The superficial lateral orbital fat compartment is located caudal to the inferior temporal septum.

The vasculature of the upper brow has been described three-dimensionally by stereoradiography using barium injection into the arterial tree. Both the superficial and the deep arteries run along a septum contiguous with the membranous boundary of the orbital retaining ligament and traverse superficially to skin, piercing the palpebral orbicularis oris oculi muscle of the upper lid. This superficial septation is perceptible during cannula-based volumizing procedures.

The sentinel vein drains into the middle temporal vein, which resides within the temporal fat pad straddled by the deep temporal fascia. The location of the supraorbital and supratrochlear neurovascular bundles is well described and familiar to most clinicians. Blindness has occurred with both injectable fillers and fat grafting procedures. The arterial diameter of both the superficial and deep arteries in the lateral brow makes intra-arterial injection only with the smallest gauge needles a possibility. However, as injection proceeds medially, arterial diameter rapidly enlarges, making small gauge needle injections significantly more risky.

Injection Pearl

During lower temporal injections, avoid the junction of the facial nerve and the anterior branch of the STA.

Fig. 4.3 illustrates the superficial temporal fat compartments.

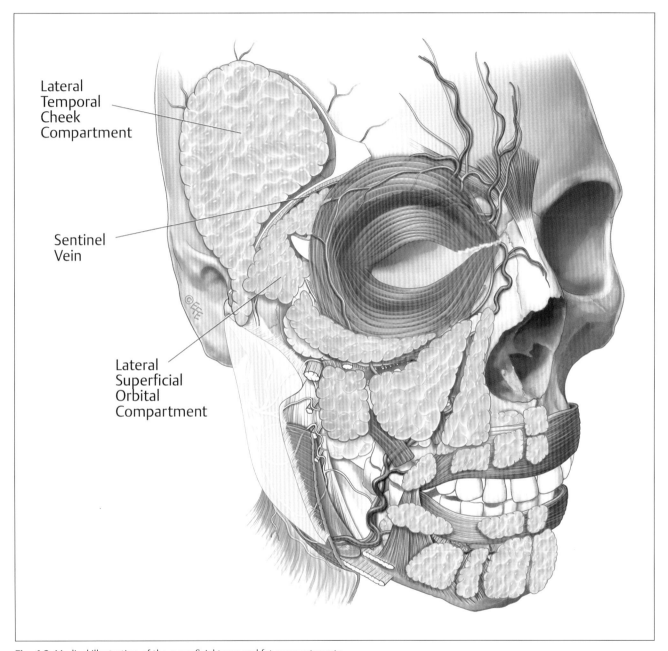

Lateral
Temporal
Cheek
Compartment

Sentinel
Vein

Lateral
Superficial
Orbital
Compartment

Fig. 4.3 Medical illustration of the superficial temporal fat compartments.

The Authors' Preferred Techniques for Temporal Volumization

Lateral Temporal (Superficial)

The insertion site for the cannula is located along the anterior border of the sideburn, 2 to 3 cm superior to the helical root. Once deep to the dermis, the cannula remains in the superficial fat and is advanced medially, the injector will feel a small amount of resistance as the cannula traverses within the fat compartment. Cannula depositions can be performed in a retrograde fanning fashion until desired aesthetic effect is achieved.

Anterior Temporal (Superficial)

The entry port is at the vertical and horizontal intersection of the sideburn. The cannula will travel on the anterior-inferior side of the superficial inferior temporal septum. This topographically correlates with Pitanguy's line. The cannula will meet resistance along the cephalad border of the space at the temporal crest. Caudally, the bounds will be the anterior two-thirds of the zygomatic arch.

Fig. 4.4 illustrates these superficial and deep temporal volumization techniques.

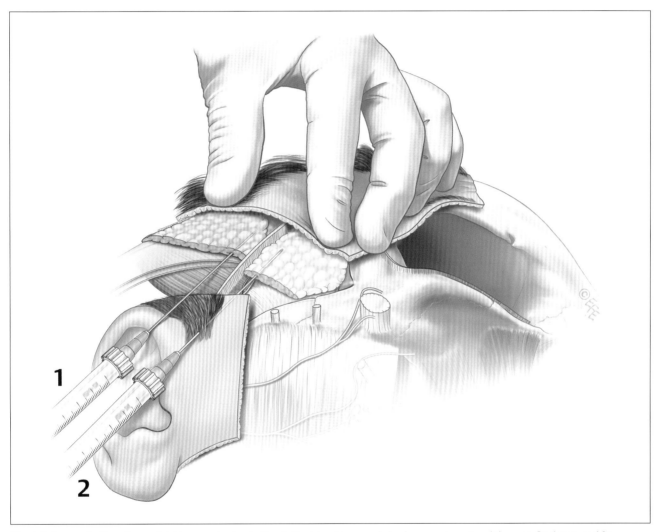

Fig. 4.4 Demonstration of superficial temporal volumization in the lateral temporal cheek compartment and the superficial temporal fat.

Deep Periorbital

Volumization of the ROOF compartment in the aging face can improve periorbital shape and appearance (**Video 4.2**). Prior to injection, the injector should attempt to palpate the supraorbital notch. This is a medial boundary and all injections should remain lateral to this boundary to avoid vascular injury. Topographic identification of the estimated location of the supraorbital and supratrochlear vessels is recommended prior to injection. The injector performs a pinch-and-pull technique of the eyebrow tissues. The needle or cannula is inserted lateral to the tail of the eyebrow and advanced medially in a deep plane cephalic to the supraorbital rim. Retrograde injection is performed until desired aesthetic effect is achieved.

Anterior Temporal

Arthur Swift has described a "1 up and 1 over" technique for anterior deep temporal volumization (**Video 4.3**). Swift states the anterior branch of the deep temporal it is no more anterior than

1.8cm from the lateral orbital rim. The injector can palpate the topography of the temple fusion line along with the scaphoid temporal fossa. The target area is 1 cm superior to supraorbital rim along the temporal fusion line and 1 cm lateral from the fusion line within the temporal fossa. This location is medial to any large temporal vasculature and deep injection should be safe from vascular injury. The injector should use a product of high G-prime and cohesivity. Prior to injection in the targeted site, the injector can feel for a pulse with digital pressure to ensure there is not a vessel traversing across the target zone. The injector will place the needle deep onto bone. At this level, the needle resides in an avascular plane, with the intent of the filler to spread between deep temporal fascia and the temporalis muscle. Prior to depositing the bolus, the injector can place the index finger of the contralateral hand on the temple hairline to prevent spread of the filler into the temple fossa underneath the hairline, thereby maximizing filler distribution in the more visible portions of the temporal fossa.

The "1 up and 1 over" technique is shown in **Fig. 4.5**.

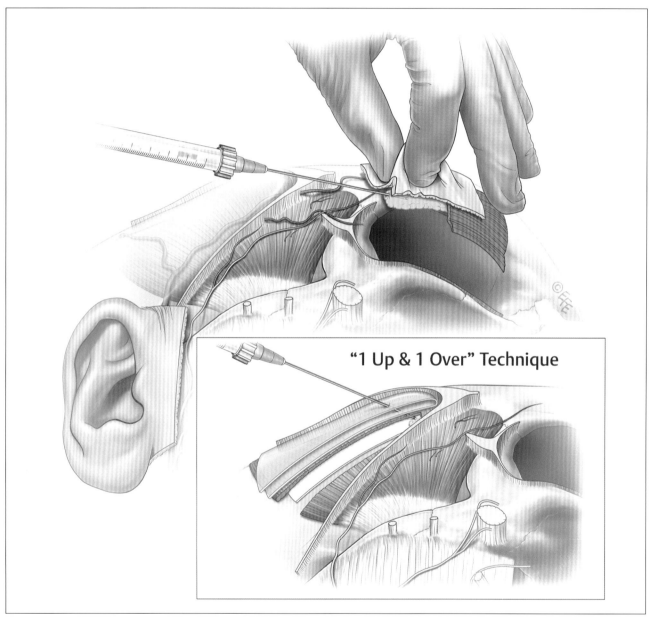

Fig. 4.5 Demonstration of anterior temporal volumization with the "1 up and 1 over" technique. Retro-orbicularis oculi fat compartment periorbital volumization is shown.

Suggested Reading

Temple Anatomy

Kawai K, Imanishi N, Nakajima H, Aiso S, Kakibuchi M, Hosokawa K. Arterial anatomical features of the upper palpebra. Plast Reconstr Surg 2004;113(2):479–484

Mendelson B, Wong C. Anatomy of the aging face. In: Neligan PC, ed. Plastic Surgery. Vol. 2. 3rd Philadelphia, PA: Elsevier Saunders; 2013:78–92

Moss CJ, Mendelson BC, Taylor GI. Surgical anatomy of the ligamentous attachments in the temple and periorbital regions. Plast Reconstr Surg 2000;105(4):1475–1490, discussion 1491–1498

O'Brien JX, Ashton MW, Rozen WM, Ross R, Mendelson BC. New perspectives on the surgical anatomy and nomenclature of the temporal region: literature review and dissection study. Plast Reconstr Surg 2013;131(3):510–522. Discussion by Knize D. on 523–525

Pessa J, Rohrich R. Facial Topography: Clinical Anatomy of the Face. St. Louis, MO: Quality Medical Publishing; 2012

Stuzin JM, Wagstrom L, Kawamoto HK, Wolfe SA. Anatomy of the frontal branch of the facial nerve: the significance of the temporal fat pad. Plast Reconstr Surg 1989;83(2):265–271

Temple Volumization and Augmentation

Fontdevila J, Serra-Renom JM, Raigosa M, et al. Assessing the long-term viability of facial fat grafts: an objective measure using computed tomography. Aesthet Surg J 2008;28(4):380–386

Gordon CR, Yaremchuk MJ. Temporal augmentation with methyl methacrylate. Aesthet Surg J 2011;31(7):827–833

Sykes JM. Applied anatomy of the temporal region and forehead for injectable fillers. J Drugs Dermatol 2009; 8(10, Suppl):s24–s27

Sykes JM, Cotofana S, Trevidic P, et al. Upper face: clinical anatomy and regional approaches with injectable fillers. Plast Reconstr Surg 2015; 136(5, Suppl):204S–218S

Index

Note: Page numbers followed by *f* or *t* indicate figures or tables, respectively.